"Every vegan, semi-vegan, or plant-based indiv...
thoughtful, thorough, game-char...
—**EVANNA LYNCH,** vegan activist and actress in

# THE *Joyful* VEGAN

How to Stay
Vegan in a World
That Wants You to
Eat Meat, Dairy,
and Eggs

# Colleen Patrick-Goudreau

Author of *The 30-Day Vegan Challenge*

# Praise for *The Joyful Vegan*

"*The Joyful Vegan* is a breath of fresh air in a world that, far too often, thumbs its nose at people who prioritize compassion. Every vegan, semi-vegan, or plant-based individual needs a copy of this thoughtful, thorough, game-changing book!"

—Evanna Lynch, vegan activist and actress in the Harry Potter film series

"*The Joyful Vegan* resonates deeply with me. Colleen Patrick-Goudreau identifies exactly what we need more of in our interactions with one another: greater empathy, understanding, and respect for our common humanity."

—Cory Booker, US senator

"Colleen Patrick-Goudreau has a unique ability to communicate with conviction and moral clarity while also acknowledging the gray areas of ethical living. With *The Joyful Vegan,* she gives voice to the universal challenges vegans face while empowering us with exactly what we need to overcome them. This book is a game-changer for new and veteran vegans alike."

—Gene Baur, president and cofounder of Farm Sanctuary and author of *Farm Sanctuary*

"This book is essential reading for anyone who has ever thought they had to choose between living ethically, eating healthfully, and engaging socially. *The Joyful Vegan* normalizes a compassionate way of living and empowers readers to embrace their values with confidence and joy."

—Kathy Freston, *New York Times* bestselling author of *Veganist*, *The Lean*, and *Clean Protein*

"Enjoying delicious, nutritious, plant-based food is easy! It's everything else that tests the most committed among us: the social pressure to conform, the emotional interactions with loved ones, and the awareness of all the unnecessary suffering. Luckily, Colleen equips us with everything we need to face these hurdles with strength and grace—and reminds us all that eating vegan is something to celebrate!"

—Michael Greger, MD, founder of NutritionFacts.org and *New York Times* bestselling author of *How Not to Die*

"By adeptly putting into words exactly what we all experience—whether we stop eating meat, dairy, and eggs for health or ethical reasons—*The Joyful Vegan* is a life-saver—literally."

—Miyoko Schinner, founder and CEO of Miyoko's, author, and activist

"The unique contribution of *The Joyful Vegan* is Colleen Patrick-Goudreau's 10 Stages that many vegans experience when they stop eating animals. The insights she provides around this concept are deeply empowering and validating for vegans who struggle living in a dominant, animal-eating culture."

—Melanie Joy, PhD, author of *Beyond Beliefs* and *Why We Love Dogs, Eat Pigs, and Wear Cows*

"With keen insights into our cultural norms and social customs, Colleen Patrick-Goudreau cements veganism and plant-based living as legitimate, healthful, and pleasurable."

—Bruce Friedrich, coauthor of *Clean Protein* and
executive director of the Good Food Institute

"In this engaging page-turner, Colleen Patrick-Goudreau draws you into her world of compassion in order to make your world better. Her skill as a writer, her purity as an observer, and her ability to make being vegan both profound and joyful will prompt you to follow her guidance and insight—whether you've been vegan for a day or for a lifetime."

—Victoria Moran, author of *Main Street Vegan* and
director, Main Street Vegan Academy

"Millions of people are going vegan. But how and why are they staying vegan? In *The Joyful Vegan*, Colleen Patrick-Goudreau examines this and more, sharing insights and tips for anyone jumping into—or considering—a vegan lifestyle. This thought-provoking and encouraging book is a must-have for anyone who aspires to go vegan and wants to *stay* vegan."

—Kristie Middleton, author of *MeatLess: Transform the
Way You Eat and Live—One Meal at a Time*

"Being vegan is about cultivating the compassion inherent in each of us. No one exemplifies this positive message better than Colleen Patrick-Goudreau, whose *Joyful Vegan* is a joy to read because of its clarion call to each of us. Her message is simple: We can each be a shining light of compassion in a world always in need of kindness."

—Toni Okamoto, author of *Plant-Based on a Budget*

"*The Joyful Vegan* is destined to be at the top of the reading list for everyone who aspires to live—and eat—consciously. The passion and authenticity of Colleen Patrick-Goudreau's book are present in every single passage. As you read, you hear Patrick-Goudreau's voice—and the clarity and logic of her expression—that make you think, 'Of course! Why didn't I think of saying it like that?' This book delivers the confidence, language, and insights you need to expand compassionate living—in your own life and in the world. Brilliant."

—Lani Muelrath, author of *The Mindful Vegan* and *The Plant-Based Journey*

"Reading *The Joyful Vegan* will help you find a compassionate and rational voice for your passion. I'm grateful to Colleen Patrick-Goudreau for helping us become better advocates for animals. Indispensable reading!"

—Tobias Leenaert, author of *How to Create a Vegan World*
and cofounder of Proveg International

# THE
## *Joyful*
# VEGAN

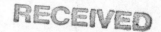

# Other Books by Colleen Patrick-Goudreau

*The Joy of Vegan Baking: More than 150 Traditional Treats and Sinful Sweets*

*The Vegan Table: 200 Unforgettable Recipes for Entertaining Every Guest at Every Occasion*

*Color Me Vegan: Maximize Your Nutrient Intake and Optimize Your Health by Eating Antioxidant-Rich, Fiber-Packed, Color-Intense Meals That Taste Great*

*Vegan's Daily Companion: 365 Days of Inspiration for Cooking, Eating, and Living Compassionately*

*The Daily Vegan: A Guided Journal,* adapted from *Vegan's Daily Companion*

*On Being Vegan: Reflections on a Compassionate Life*

*The 30-Day Vegan Challenge: The Ultimate Guide to Eating Healthfully and Living Compassionately*

# THE

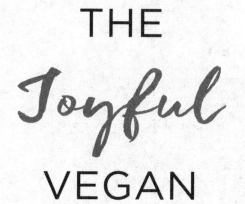

*Joyful*

# VEGAN

## How to Stay Vegan in a World That Wants You to Eat Meat, Dairy, and Eggs

COLLEEN PATRICK-GOUDREAU

BenBella Books, Inc.
Dallas, Texas

BenBella Books, Inc.
10440 N. Central Expressway, Suite 800
Dallas, TX 75231
www.benbellabooks.com
Send feedback to feedback@benbellabooks.com

Printed in the United States of America
10 9 8 7 6 5 4 3 2 1

Library of Congress Cataloging-in-Publication Data: 2019015072
ISBN 9781948836463 (trade cloth)
ISBN 9781948836715 (ebook)

Editing by Leah Wilson
Copyediting by Karen Wise
Proofreading by James Fraleigh and Cape Cod Compositors, Inc.
Text design and composition by PerfecType, Nashville, TN
Cover design by Oceana Garaceau
Cover photo by Connie Pugh and iStock / alicjane
Author photo by Michelle Cehn
Printed by Lake Book Manufacturing

Distributed to the trade by Two Rivers Distribution, an Ingram brand
www.tworiversdistribution.com

Special discounts for bulk sales are available.
Please contact bulkorders@benbellabooks.com.

*To David*

*You are my heart, my soul, and my rock. You inspire me to be a better person every day and beautifully model what it means to be a joyful vegan.*

# CONTENTS

Introduction   |   1
*The Making of a Joyful Vegan*

## Section One   Becoming Vegan

### Chapter One

"Don't Tell Me. I Don't Want to Know"   |   15
*Blissful Ignorance and Willful Blindness*

### Chapter Two

The Awakening   |   39
*The Epiphany That Changes Everything*

## Section Two   Staying Vegan

### Stage One

Bearing Witness   |   61
*Compassion Fatigue, Self-Care, and the
Voracious Consumption of Information*

## Stage Two
### Guilt, Regret, and Remorse | 85
*Finding Peace and Choosing Self-Forgiveness*

## Stage Three
### Coming Out Vegan | 105
*Explaining the V-Word to Family,
Friends, and Yourself*

## Stage Four
### Evangelism and Fundamentalism | 135
*Knowing the Difference Between Enthusiasm
and Zealotry*

## Stage Five
### The Angry Vegan | 149
*Dispelling the Stereotype and
Understanding Its Roots*

## Stage Six
### Finding Your Tribe | 163
*Embracing Your Identity, Building Community,
and Feeling a Sense of Belonging*

## Stage Seven
### Finding Your Voice | 189
*How to Talk to a Hunter
(Or Anyone Else with Whom You Disagree)*

*Stage Eight*

**Stretching Your Comfort Zones** | 211
*Expansion of Awareness and Skills*

*Stage Nine*

**Finding Your Place** | 223
*Advocacy and Activism*

*Stage Ten*

**Integration and Adaptation** | 263
*Identifying as a Joyful Vegan
in a Nonvegan World*

Acknowledgments | 271

Special Recognition | 273

Resources and Recommendations | 275

Endnotes | 279

About the Author | 289

# INTRODUCTION

# The Making of a Joyful Vegan

> My doctrine is this, that if we see cruelty or wrong
> that we have the power to stop, and do nothing,
> we make ourselves sharers in the guilt.
> —Anna Sewell, *Black Beauty*

I was raised in a typical American family eating typical American fare: pretty much anything that came from an animal who had once walked, swum, or flown. Nightly dinners in our Irish-American home consisted of a rotation of pork chops, lamb stew, meatloaf, veal cutlets, and ground beef, along with some token vegetables on the side, always slathered with butter or submerged in cream-based sauces. With a father who owned ice cream shops and who kept a separate freezer just to store the gallons of frozen treats he brought home, I enjoyed dairy-rich desserts on a daily basis. We had a milkshake machine, a hot chocolate maker, and more candy than Willy Wonka would know what to do with. There was no dearth of animal products in our home, and I ate them all with fervor.

I was also a typical child in that I cared about animals. I'm reluctant to say I "loved animals," because I don't believe you have to love animals to not want to hurt them, but I did (and do) *adore* animals. I've always loved being around them, I've never had a fear of them, and I shed tears at the slightest hint of them suffering at all—in real life or in books, television shows, or movies. When I was eight years old, a bird with an injured wing fell from a tree in our yard, so I built a little house for her until she was well enough to fly again. When stray dogs made their way to our doorstep, I brought them in until I could return them to their homes. When my mother took me to see *Benji*—a film about a homeless dog who endures hunger, abuse, and loneliness before endearing himself to a human family—she had to drag me out of the theatre mid-film for all of my weeping and wailing.

> You don't have to *love* animals to *not* want to hurt them.

I remember the day we adopted our own dog, Charmaine, an adorable, tiny gray schnauzer with floppy ears and a loud, persistent bark. She whimpered incessantly the first few nights she was with us, which tormented me greatly. This in turn tormented my mother, who would find me in tears at her bedside in the middle of the night begging to let our puppy come to bed with me so I could soothe her to sleep. My mother relented, and we all enjoyed restful nights thereafter. The emotional attachment I had to that little dog (and her to me) was gravely underestimated by my parents a few years later when, during a painful divorce and custody battle, she was taken from me with no warning. I was able to see her periodically, and eventually as a young adult I was able to arrange to have her live with me again, but the memory of the loss of that daily bond still stings.

My empathy for animals has always run quite deep, but I don't think my affection for them was very different from that of most children.

Parents, teachers, and adults in general foster a connection between children and animals from the time we're born—evidenced by everything from the clothes they dress us in and the books they read to us to the movies they screen for us and the songs they teach us. Most of us had images of baby animals adorning our childhood clothing, wallpaper, and bedding; animal cutouts hung over our cribs in a musical mobile; and plush animals that served as our constant companions. As children, we're taught songs about animals and play games where we imitate animals; we're brought to the zoo to admire animals; and on Halloween, many of us dress up as our favorite animal. (Many of us still do as adults.) More than that, the adults around us use animals (albeit fictional ones) to teach us our most fundamental skills: how to count, how to spell, how to read, and how to talk.

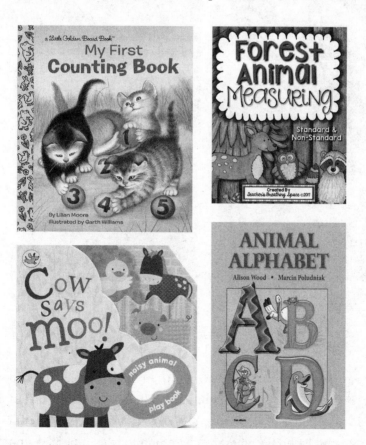

Through allegories and fables—both ancient and modern—animals even help shape our mental character by teaching us social mores, proper manners, and moral conduct. A methodical tortoise taught me that slow and steady wins the race, a panicked chicken taught me not to jump to conclusions even if the sky appears to be falling, and three bears—a mama, a papa, and a baby—highlighted just how annoying little girls can be and how rude it is to intrude upon animals in their homes. (At least, that was *my* takeaway. I may have missed the point of that one.)

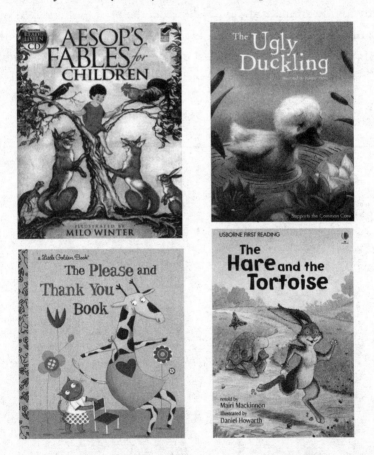

Many stories we read as children are written expressly for the purpose of raising awareness about the plight and welfare of animals, including such classics as *Bambi*, *Black Beauty*, and *Charlotte's Web*, and often it's a large-hearted child who becomes the champion for the imperiled animal, reflecting back to our impressionable minds a model for human–animal relations. Although the Disneyfied adaptations tend to dilute some of the poignancy of the original texts, the films still leave deep impressions on many of us. Who among us remained unmoved when Bambi learns his mother was killed by hunters or when Dumbo's mother strains to rock her baby through the bars that imprison her? Or when Black Beauty is passed from one cruel owner to the next? *Charlotte's Web* is the reason many children stop eating pigs, and despite its sixty-plus years, it continues to inspire many to become vegetarian—or to at least take a step toward that end. Jack London's *Call of the Wild*, about a dog stolen from his home to be sold into service as a sled dog, still leaves an indelible impression upon students who read it in school. And Winnie the Pooh, along with his legion of furry pals, remains a link to the best parts of our childhood, when life was simple and our best friends were talking animals.

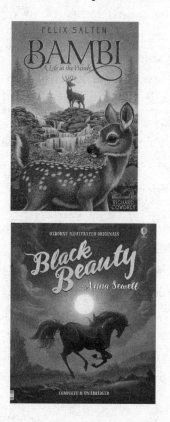
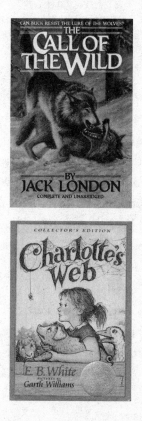

Granted, I'm speaking of characters in fiction and film, but the relationships (or lack thereof) we have with animals as children in many ways shape who we become as adults—as human beings. More than that, they *reflect* who we are as humans. How children relate to animals is often used as a barometer for determining mental or emotional health. We know that if a child is kind to an animal, it's a good sign. It demonstrates that the child is capable of tenderness, compassion, attachment, and empathy. On the other hand, if a child abuses or hurts an animal, it's considered a red flag. The National School Safety Council, the US Department of Education, the American Psychological Association, and the National Crime Prevention Council all agree that animal cruelty is a strong predictor of potential violence against humans.[1] In other words, the research bears out what we know instinctively and anecdotally: that the more children are encouraged to bond with animals, the more they experience empathy and exhibit compassion—for everyone, humans and nonhumans alike.

> The relationships we have with animals as children shape who we become as adults and reflect who we are as human beings.

My parents, teachers, and other adults in my life didn't necessarily know about this research, yet in practically every aspect of my life I was encouraged to have a relationship with animals and was given the message that nonhuman animals were integral to who I was—and helping to shape who I was becoming. What I didn't know was that, at the same time, I was being fed the dismembered bodies of animals—animals no different from the ones I was brought to the zoo to pet or whose wings I helped mend or whose likenesses ornamented my pajamas and lunchbox. And so I was taught—implicitly, of course—to categorize animals into arbitrary compartments of those we care for and those we eat, those we live with and those we exploit, those worthy of our compassion and those undeserving of it simply because they happen to be of a particular species or bred for a particular use. In other words: *puppies* good, *calves* food. (But only *some* puppies, as we'll explore in a subsequent chapter.)

The message I received by the time I was old enough to understand I was eating animals was that the injured bird who was lucky enough to fall into my yard was worth saving, but the chickens and turkeys who "sacrificed themselves so I could eat" were valuable only in so far as their flesh was tender and juicy. In other words: *chickadees* friends, *chickens* dinner. This arbitrary distinction makes our consumption of them possible, but to animals, it's all the same. To paraphrase the late Broadway actress and animal activist Gretchen Wyler: If they have wings, they want to fly. If they have legs, they want to walk. If they have voices, they want to communicate. If they have offspring, they want to nurture them. Having lives, they want to keep them. But these are choices we have taken from animals. That is our legacy. Animals are not the masters of their own fate or freedom. We are.

At the same time I was subconsciously learning to categorize animals, I was also learning to compartmentalize and temper my own compassion. In response to any questions I posed about what (or who) I was eating and why, I was given the message that life is not always fair and nature is not always kind, but God put animals on Earth for us to eat and I should be grateful for His kindness and their sacrifice. (I was raised in a Catholic/Protestant home, but the idea that humans are the overlords of other animals is indubitably universal and ecumenical, subscribed to by atheists and believers alike.) As a result, that fierce, unconditional compassion I had as a child began to dull, as my taste for animal flesh, fat, and fluids began to grow and settle into my palate.

> If they have wings, they want to fly. If they have legs, they want to walk. If they have offspring, they want to nurture them.

I continued to devour all manner of fried legs, barbecued ribs, smoked backs, breaded wings, boiled eggs, flavored fluids, and whatever else came off of or out of an animal. I wore leather, wool, fur, and cashmere, slept under down comforters, and even tried my hand at fishing and falconry. I'd like to say I gave no thought to the animals whose flesh and secretions I was consuming, but that wouldn't be entirely true. Like most people, I ate what was socially acceptable and culturally palatable, and was viscerally disgusted at the thought of eating gizzards, livers, hearts, or feet—or dogs, cats, or horses. As I grew older, I internalized the narrative that "animals are here for us" and that "cows need to be milked for their own good," and I trusted the marketing terms ("free-range," "organic," "humane") that enabled me to justify my consumption of animals while mitigating any guilt I may have harbored. I also never fished again, because I'd seen what it looked like for an animal to die; during all the years I was eating animals, of course I never wanted to actually see how they were killed.

And then some light began to appear through the cracks of my protective shell. When I was about twenty years old, I read *Diet for a New America* by John Robbins, and the course of my life changed forever. This was one of the first books to examine the effects of an animal-based diet on our health, on the environment, and on animals themselves, and it was certainly the first time I had ever seen the images of animal factories, where lives are regarded as machines and the value of animals is determined only by what and how much their bodies can produce. I couldn't take my eyes off the photos of hens in cages with the tips of their beaks seared off, female "breeding" pigs confined in crates the size of their own overgrown bodies, turkeys packed in windowless sheds, and calves chained to boxes. I remember staring at those images in disbelief. How could I not have known about this? How could I have contributed to it? How could this even happen? I knew right away that I didn't want to be part of it, so I stopped eating land animals that very day.

Interestingly, my parents—and others—didn't quite react the same way they had when I was a child. Helping fallen baby birds or taking in stray animals were considered admirable childhood pursuits and met with support and admiration, but when that very same compassion—though no different in substance or strength—followed me into adulthood and extended to pigs, cattle, chickens, and other animals brought into this world only to be killed, it was greeted with hostility and suspicion. The message was: *Limited compassion* good, *unconditional compassion* bad. *Childhood compassion* normal, *adult compassion* excessive. Despite the fact that compassion is a guiding principle in all the world's religions and most secular philosophies, the primary message we receive by the time we're adults is that compassion is conditional—reserved only for certain groups/species. And though we appreciate and even admire compassion in children, we're taught to be somewhat suspicious of compassion in adults, deeming it sentimental and irrational. Operating within these boundaries of selective compassion, how can we not feel a weight on our minds and a heaviness in our hearts?

Nonetheless, my awakening had begun, and I was not deterred. I was, however, still partially asleep. I had stopped eating land animals, was learning everything I could about issues related to our food system, and had begun advocating for animals through education and outreach, but I continued to consume chicken's eggs, cow's milk, and aquatic animals. This lasted for several years until I was knocked into full consciousness while reading *Slaughterhouse: The Shocking Story of Greed, Neglect, and Inhumane Treatment Inside the U.S. Meat Industry* by investigative journalist Gail Eisnitz. I have never forgotten how painful it was to read this book and how powerful it was to feel my eyes and heart opening. Becoming fully awake was a visceral, harrowing process, but I wouldn't change it for all the world—however many tears I shed in the few days it took me to read the book. The lens through which I saw the world completely changed, and the paradigm by which I lived my life totally shifted.

I came to fully comprehend that no matter how an animal is "raised" or what he or she is "raised for" (flesh, eggs, or milk), in the end, it's all the same, and that end is characterized by violence. After reading *Diet for a New America*, I would have said that I stopped eating land animals because I didn't like the way they were treated. But after reading

*Slaughterhouse*, it became much more fundamental than that. I became aware of how wasteful, unnecessary, and absurd it is to bring animals into this world only to kill them; I became disgusted at how we manipulate the reproductive system of females for their milk, capitalizing on their ability to give birth only to take their young from them and impregnate them again and again and again. I became fully cognizant of the violence inherent in breeding, keeping, transporting, and killing animals for our pleasure and wholly uncomfortable that I was complicit in paying people to become desensitized to their own compassion as well as to animal suffering. I realized I was supporting a culture of violence whose consequences are incalculable and permanent, which didn't sit well with me. I felt as if I had been sleepwalking up until that moment. Now that I was awake, I couldn't help but act. My natural response was to stop participating in this system, and so, still reeling from what I was reading, I called my soon-to-be-husband and told him: "I'm becoming vegan."

I'm struck by how funny that phrase can sound. We say a caterpillar "becomes" a butterfly or a seed "becomes" a flower and can easily imagine what they look like before and after their transformation. But what does it look like to *become* vegan? What did I *become* when I *became vegan*? Was there really a difference between the *pre-vegan* me and the *post-vegan* me? Prior to *being vegan*, I considered myself a compassionate person living a compassionate life—even advocating for animals in my way. But, in truth, my actions were not fully in alignment with my self-perception. In truth, I was not *really* living my life according to my deepest values—the values I've held dear since I was a child and that defined me as a person. I would never have intentionally hurt another living being, yet I was paying others to do it for me. Reading the personal accounts of slaughterhouse workers who abused, dismembered, tortured, and killed animals as a matter of routine shook me to my core and out of my slumber.

*Becoming vegan* was my metamorphosis into unconditional, unfettered, unabashed compassion. That is to say, when I *became vegan*, my deepest ethics became reflected in my daily choices, and the process was as natural and effortless as is the process for a caterpillar becoming a butterfly or a seed becoming a flower. Of course, births—and rebirths—are also messy and painful and not without their challenges, but they're always worth the trouble in the end.

Before I became vegan, I was unaware of the ways in which I contributed to violence against animals. Once I knew, I couldn't unknow. And I had to act. I chose—and continue to choose—to remain aware, awake, and engaged. There are many forces out there that compel us to revert to our old ways of thinking and behaving, and none of us are impervious to that pressure. It is for that reason I wrote this book: to link my story with yours, to guide you on your own journey of awakening, and to create a roadmap to help you stay the course, even as you encounter bumps, blocks, barricades, and booby traps along the way.

> When I *became vegan*, my deepest ethics became reflected in my daily choices.

*The Joyful Vegan* is our collective story—of how we got to where we are, and how to keep going forward with conviction and joy.

Section One

# BECOMING VEGAN

efore I knew, I didn't know. Once I did, everything changed.

I've heard enough origin stories—stories of how people became vegan or plant-based—to know how alike they all are. Of course, the particulars are unique, but at the center of all our stories is that we *stopped knowing*—willingly, if unwittingly. *Unwittingly* because we don't know we're unconscious until we come to; we don't know we're asleep until we wake up. *Willingly* because, even while sleeping, a part of us knows we are, in fact, asleep.

And yet, that's not where our story ends. Despite every reason to stay asleep, still we wake up. Despite the comfort of ignorant bliss, still we choose to know, to look, to change.

*Chapter One*

# "Don't Tell Me. I Don't Want to Know"

## *Blissful Ignorance and Willful Blindness*

I don't think we did go blind, I think we are blind, Blind
but seeing, Blind people who can see, but do not see.

—José Saramago, *Blindness*

When we turn away from the reality of what we do to animals
for our gustatory pleasure, how raising them harms ecosystems, and how eating them negatively affects our health, we
play a game of pretend, like the child who covers her eyes and thinks you
can't see her. And yet, there she remains. Closing our eyes and turning
away from reality doesn't make the reality disappear; it only closes our

minds and hearts and allows the reality to continue. *Don't tell me; I don't want to know. Don't show me; I don't want to look.* We sense that were we to open our eyes, we would be compelled to change, and it's change we want to avoid. *I don't want to see what takes place on dairy farms; I'd have to stop eating cheese! I don't want to know how pigs are killed; I love bacon too much!* Wary of the unknown that lies on the other side of awareness, we opt for what is familiar and secure: the certainty of denial, the comfort of willful blindness.

In her book *Willful Blindness: Why We Ignore the Obvious at Our Peril*, author Margaret Heffernan explains that the term "willful blindness" (also called "willful ignorance" or "contrived ignorance") originated in the legal profession, where it refers to "the state of mind that accompanied one who 'willfully shut his eyes' as 'connivance' or 'constructive knowledge.'"[1] It's the idea that if there's information that you *could* know or *should* know but you somehow manage *not to know*, the law determines that you're *willfully blind*—that you've *chosen* not to know. Today, willful blindness is used outside jurisprudence—its meaning has broadened to refer to any situation in which people intentionally turn away from an ethical dilemma, especially one in which they may be complicit. "Our complicity lies not in a direct infliction of violence," writes author Timothy Pachirat, author of *Every Twelve Seconds: Industrialized Slaughter and the Politics of Sight*, "but rather in our tacit agreement to look away." Look away. Turn a blind eye. Reinforced by institutional, social, commercial, and political support, willful blindness is as widespread and socially sanctioned as our consumption of animal flesh and fluids.

Institutionally, politically, and commercially, we see it in the windowless sheds in which animals are confined and concealed, in the so-called ag-gag laws that make it a crime to document the conditions of these animals, in the euphemisms that describe animals as being "harvested" and "processed" rather than "killed" and "dismembered," in the marketing terms that normalize and romanticize the consumption of animals and their offspring, in the government subsidies that favor animal agriculture and its monied lobbyists, and in the resulting biased nutrition recommendations.

Individually and socially, we see willful blindness reinforced by our desire to conform to tradition, social norms, family expectations, cultural mores, and our own perception of ourselves as compassionate and health-savvy people. We see it in the belief deeply held by meat-eaters that to eat animals is to be neutral or impartial and that to be vegan is to take a position or to "have an agenda," as if being part of the status quo precludes you from bias. But, of course, just because an idea is shared by many doesn't mean it's not an ideology or that its proponents aren't zealots. (The only reason nonvegans' irrational devotion to meat, dairy, and eggs is not seen as fanatical is that it represents the status quo.) As social psychologist Dr. Melanie Joy, author of *Why We Love Dogs, Eat Pigs, and Wear Cows,* points out, everyone "brings their beliefs and values to the dinner table"—not just vegans—and by believing that animal consumption is "normal, natural, and necessary," which Joy calls the "three N's of justification," and that veganism is *deviant* and *unnatural,* we avoid conflict and change by remaining blissfully ignorant and willfully blind.[2]

> Just because an idea is shared by many doesn't mean it's not an ideology or that its proponents aren't zealots.

It's often said that ignorance is bliss, but is it really? After all, as I experienced and described in the introduction—and as I've heard countless vegans recount in their own stories—supporting something we know to be inherently violent and undeniably painful necessitates the numbing of our compassion and the hardening of our hearts. We *have* to look away, live in ignorance, and defy our own conscience in order to partake in something that goes against some of our most intrinsic values. We *have* to create boundaries to our compassion and place animals in arbitrary categories in order to continue supporting something that is anathema to our very ethics or a threat to our well-being. Cognitive dissonance necessitates our willful blindness.

Cognitive dissonance, a term coined by social psychologist Leon Festinger in 1957, refers to the turmoil we feel when our mind tries to hold two wholly incompatible views at the same time or when we engage in behavior that conflicts with our beliefs.[3] When it comes to our consumption of animals, dissonance (i.e., conflict, tension, discord) is created when we struggle to reconcile our compassion—our desire to protect animals from harm and our belief that we're good people—with our habitual taste and preference for animal-based meat, milk, and eggs. It's incredibly difficult to hold both beliefs at the same time: that animals feel pain *and* that we're causing them to suffer, that the consumption of animal products creates disease *and* that we eat them anyway (and feed them to our loved ones). The dissonance produced by mutually exclusive beliefs is tremendously painful, even unbearable. A growing body of research that examines the psychology of eating animals offers some insight into how we cope with this tension.

> It's incredibly difficult to hold these two beliefs at the same time: that animals feel pain *and* that we're causing them to suffer.

## THE STORIES WE TELL OURSELVES

The average consumer in the United States eats more than 200 pounds of animal-based meat per year,[4] more than three times the global average.[5] We eat quantities of meat that are unprecedented in human history, and yet we clearly also care about the welfare and well-being of nonhuman animals. According to the American Pet Products Association, US households have more than 300 million companion animals, on whom we spend over $60 billion annually.[6] But it's not just companion animals—cats, dogs, rabbits, fish, and birds—we care about; Americans consistently call for protection for farmed animals as well. A 2016 survey funded by the ASPCA found that 77 percent of consumers say that they are concerned about the welfare of animals raised for human consumption,[7] and according to a national poll from 2015, 86 percent of meat-eating Americans say it's important that farmed animals be treated humanely.[8] Concern for the treatment of animals spans income level, party affiliation, sex, and race, and it's conveyed consistently in survey data going back several decades.

So, how is it that we genuinely don't want to see animals suffer and yet bring billions of them into the world each year only to kill them? How do we reconcile our compassion for their living selves with our voracious appetite for their dismembered flesh? How can we *feel* one way yet *act* in such a contradictory way?

Psychologists studying this tension have named this the "meat paradox," the phenomenon whereby "people care about animals and do not want to see them harmed but engage in a diet that requires them to be killed and, usually, to suffer."[9] As posited by the theory of cognitive dissonance, when faced with a conflict like this—when our actions don't reflect our ethics—we tend to take one of two roads:

1. We change our behavior to align with our beliefs.
2. We change our beliefs to align with our behavior.

The first plays out most obviously in the behavior of vegetarians and vegans, who choose to stop eating the flesh of animals, as well as their eggs and milk, respectively (and even in "reducetarians," who purposefully and substantially reduce their consumption of animal products). The second manifests in more subtle ways, such as changing our perception of animals themselves.

Research has found that the way we *perceive* animals is intimately tied to our ability to *eat* them; for instance, according to researchers on the psychology of meat consumption, "eating animals is morally troublesome when animals are perceived as worthy of moral concern. The more moral concern we afford an entity, the more immoral it becomes to harm it."[10] Research psychologists have found that one way of resolving the tension between our compassion for animals and our consumption of them is to categorize living animals as "food," such as when we refer to "pork" instead of "pig," "beef" instead of "cow," and "veal" instead of "calf." Psychologists posit that this "act of categorization may shift our focus away from morally relevant attributes (i.e., the capacity to suffer—mentally, emotionally, or physically), and therefore change our perception of" and our moral concern for the animal.[11] Reducing animals to inanimate objects, we resolve our cognitive dissonance not by changing our behavior to no longer cause suffering to animals, but by removing the belief that (certain) animals can and do suffer. The effect is a lessening of our ethical concern for them and a rationalizing of our consumption of them.*

> The way we *perceive* animals is intimately tied to our ability to *eat* them.

By linguistically cleaving animals into arbitrary categories—"food animals," "circus animals," "pets," "laboratory animals," "wildlife," "farm animals"—we unconsciously create differences in how we perceive and treat the animals within those categories. This is the case even when animals are part of the same species. For instance, we may accept that a dog in a laboratory will be put through agonizing procedures but agree that a dog who lives with a family in a home deserves to be protected against pain and suffering. The dog in the lab has the same capacity to suffer as the dog in the home, but our classification of one as a "laboratory subject" and the other as a "pet" enables us to rationalize our exploitation of one and our nurturing of the other.†

---

\* Please consult the Resources and Recommendations section at the back of this book for books that focus on the inner lives and intelligence of animals.

† Of course, our intimate relationship with the animals we have in our homes affects

Similarly, our treatment and slaughter of animals bred and killed for human consumption would be illegal if applied to dogs and cats. The ability to feel pain and the desire to avoid death are the same in all animals, but our subjective categorizations of them sanctions our exploitation of cows (and pigs, goats, chickens, or turkeys) and our protection of dogs and cats. This compartmentalization—and the fact that it's socially acceptable—explains why we're outraged that dogs and cats are killed for "meat" in certain countries around the world, while we have no problem with the fact that cows, pigs, goats, chickens, and turkeys are killed for the same right here at home. They are all capable of feeling pain; they are all eager to live. In these ways, they are all the same. It's our subjective *perception* of the animals—not any objective *quality* of animals—that compels us to eat one and not the other.

The social drivers that compel us to eat animals are manifold, and I'm not suggesting that simply calling the animal flesh we eat by the names of the living animals we kill would solve the problem. What I *am* saying is that these lexical distinctions help lessen our inner conflict. After all, we don't have separate lexicons for the plant foods we eat. Growing in a garden or served on a plate, a potato is still a potato. We can witness a fruit harvest with no compunction and call it what it is. There is no need to distinguish between the blossoming apple and the plucked apple. When we categorize pigs, cows, chickens, and turkeys as "food animals," we are implicitly declaring that we "don't want to look" at what happens to these animals. We are making the choice to be self-deluded, to be asleep rather than awake, to be willfully blind.*

---

our perception. Most of us have never had a turkey fall asleep on our lap, played chase with a pig, or snuggled with a cow. When we do have these experiences, we often have a change of heart about who these animals are and what they're capable of feeling. In other words, we tend to protect what we know and value.

* But what about the animals for whom we don't have separate words to distinguish between the living and the slaughtered? How do we reconcile the fact that many of us would be uneasy ordering "cow," "steer," "calf," "bull," or "ox" from a menu but are unfazed asking for a meal made with "turkey," "chicken," "rabbit," or "fish"? I have a few theories I don't have space to elaborate on here,

Contributing to violence against animals is inconsistent with who most of us are, with how we perceive ourselves, with the values most of us hold, and with the goals most of us have, but faced with the choice between continuing to delude ourselves and changing our behavior, self-delusion comes out looking pretty appealing. Change can be *very* difficult—even terrifying—evoking subconscious fears of varying rationality: fear of the unknown, fear of rocking the boat, fear of conflict, fear of being rejected, fear of disobeying. And so, if we can't or don't want to change the behavior that causes the dissonance (in other words, stop eating animal flesh and fluids), we have to change our *thinking* about the behavior; *we have to remove the dissonance.*

We are equally deluded when it comes to our denial about the detrimental health effects of consuming high amounts of meat, dairy, and eggs and low amounts of whole grains, beans, fruits, vegetables, and nuts. We clearly care about our health. A 2017 study of US adults aged eighteen to sixty-five found that the average American spends $155 per month on health and fitness, which comes to $112,000 over a lifetime.[12] Yet in one of the most technologically and medically advanced nations on the planet, we are dying from diseases that could be prevented (and reversed) by simple changes in diet and lifestyle. Decades of research and peer-reviewed studies unequivocally conclude that our poor diet is the number one cause of premature death and the number one cause of disability in the United States.[13]

---

but cultural and personal conditioning plays a role; we're taught from a young age to use the word "beef" to refer to the flesh of cattle, "pork" to refer to the flesh of pigs, and "chicken" to refer to the flesh of chickens. Over the hundreds of years we've been using "chicken" and "turkey," for instance, to refer to the meat of these animals, we've stripped them of their once-living sources. Saying "chicken" to denote the flesh of that animal has become as removed from the living chicken as "beef" has from "cow." However, by making a simple semantic tweak, such as referring to eating "chickens" (rather than "chicken") and "turkeys" (rather than "turkey"), a lifeless slab of meat gets transformed in our minds into squawking, feathered birds.

It's not just individual spending habits that reveal this dissonance. As a nation, the United States spends 18 percent of its annual gross domestic product on health, which in 2015 amounted to $3.2 trillion.[14] Yet despite such a rich investment, American health is, by most standards of measurement, worse than that of any other wealthy nation. So how is it that we genuinely care about our health and yet participate in behaviors that are antithetical to attaining that health? How do we reconcile our desire to thrive with our voracious appetite for products that contribute to disease? How can we *feel* one way yet *act* in such a contradictory way?

Just as we resolve our ethical quandary about eating animals by changing our perception of the animals raised and killed for our consumption, denying their ability to suffer, and undermining the trauma they experience when their babies are taken from them or when they're perpetually confined in cages and crates, so too do we resolve our concerns about unhealthful foods and eating habits by changing our *minds*—rather than our *behavior*. One way we do this is by downplaying or dismissing the research that confirms the negative effects of eating meat, dairy, and eggs; we do this whether we're talking about the effects on animals, on the environment, or on our health. We also cherry-pick which data we want to believe depending on how well it supports or opposes our ideology or perspective.

- *The research that says eggs are bad for you is inconclusive. I just don't believe it.*
- *Studies contradict themselves all the time. One day it's harmful to eat meat; the next day it's the best thing for us. It's too confusing, so I just eat what I want.*
- *If eating animal products was so harmful, the government and health officials would never allow it.*
- *Heart disease and diabetes run in my family. My genes have already predisposed me to disease, so it doesn't matter what I eat.*
- *My grandfather ate cheese, butter, and cream sauces every day and lived to be ninety-five, so clearly they can't be bad for you.*

- *I buy only "organic" meat/dairy/eggs, which don't have the same environmental impacts as conventionally raised versions; in fact, studies show that organic animal products are environmentally friendly.*
- *I buy milk from "happy cows," who are treated very well.*

Another way we resolve our internal conflict is to reduce or subvert the importance of our own values and beliefs.

- *Of course I care about animals, but I just love cheese so much.*
- *I know pigs are more intelligent than dogs and don't deserve to be abused or killed, but I could never live without bacon.*
- *Hurting animals goes against everything I believe, but life is short. We should enjoy what we can while we're alive.*
- *Of course my children love animals, but it's more important that they fit in and not be ostracized for being vegetarian/vegan, so I feed them meat.*
- *I'd rather be vegetarian/vegan—I even tried it once—but my doctor/ naturopath/nutritionist/acupuncturist told me I need to eat meat.*
- *I don't want to eat meat, but my blood type says I'm supposed to.*

Of course we should rely on science and trusted professionals to help make decisions about our health, but we should also make sure we're not simply looking for "experts" who will confirm our bias and "gurus" who will tell us what we want to hear. In his book, *States of Denial: Knowing About Atrocities and Suffering*, author Stanley Cohen identifies *obedience to superiors* as one of the ways we deny responsibility for harmful actions.[15] We see this deference to authority in the last two bullet points—when we say we eat animal products "because my doctor told me to" (despite the fact that fewer than 20 percent of medical schools have a single required course in nutrition)* or because we're conditioned to believe that "milk

---

* Doctors are trusted and influential sources for many people, who value their opinion even if it's just that. Most medical doctors don't have training in nutrition, but according to the International Food Information Council's 2018 Food and Health Survey, 78 percent of individuals say they make changes in their eating

does a body good" (even though that information came to us from biased advertisements benefiting the dairy industry) or because "eating meat is sanctioned in the Bible" (even though eating a plant-based diet is espoused in one section of the Bible* and eating pigs, for example, is forbidden in another†). I've heard from countless individuals who tell me they genuinely want to be vegan/vegetarian but feel they can't because their doctor/religion/parents/some authority figure told them they can't or shouldn't. In order to minimize discomfort without the inconvenience of making behavioral changes, we relinquish our own agency and discernment and instead submit to the wishes and opinions of others—even though we should know that they're biased.

*Don't tell me how bad this burger is; I don't want to know. Don't show me how animals are treated; I don't want to look. Don't tell my children where the meat they eat comes from. It would upset them too much.* When there is dissonance, not only do we try to reduce it, we also "actively avoid situations and information which would likely increase the dissonance," posited Festinger.[16] As a result, most of us completely avoid looking at the things that would cause us the most pain and the most dissonance: the slaughter of animals or the evidence that implicates meat, dairy, and eggs in our ailments and illnesses. As Festinger and other scholars such as *Willful Blindness* author Margaret Heffernan argued, "We all strive to preserve an image of ourselves as consistent, stable, competent, and good.

---

habits as a result of conversations with their doctors. Of course this is problematic when these recommendations are based on personal bias or old information, such as "eat more white meat" or "the fat in eggs is good for you, but cut down on olive oil." See https://foodinsight.org/wp-content/uploads/2018/05/2018-FHS-Report-FINAL.pdf.

\* The Bible explains God's original will in Genesis 1:29–30: "Then God said, 'I give you every seed-bearing plant on the face of the whole earth and every tree that has fruit with seed in it. They will be yours for food. And to all the beasts of the earth and all the birds in the sky and all the creatures that move along the ground—everything that has the breath of life in it—I give every green plant for food.'"

† Leviticus 11:7–8 states, "And the pig, because it parts the hoof and is cloven-footed but does not chew the cud, is unclean to you. You shall not eat any of their flesh, and you shall not touch their carcasses; they are unclean to you."

We simply could not function if we believed ourselves to be otherwise. Our most cherished beliefs are a vital and central part of who we are—in our own eyes and in the eyes of our friends and colleagues. And so we strive mightily to reduce the pain, either by ignoring the evidence that proves we are wrong, or by reinterpreting evidence to support us."[17] Fear of conflict, fear of change, fear of not fitting in compels us to do so.

But more than just ignoring or reinterpreting the evidence, we even go so far as to reframe our harmful choices as both *necessary* and *beneficial*.

> In order to protect our sense of ourselves as good people, we reframe transgressive behaviors as noble ones.

In order to protect our sense of ourselves as good people, we have to reframe any transgressions that would contradict that. In order to preserve our sense of self-worth when we participate in harmful behaviors, we have to transform those behaviors into noble ones. We not only defend our exploitation of animals for food, fun, or fashion by asserting that it's economically necessary and biologically/ nutritionally essential for us ("we can't live without animal protein," "we need meat to survive," "ranchers would be unemployed if we stopped eating meat," etc.), we also assert that it's beneficial for the animals—even the very animals we bring into this world only to kill.

- *By killing animals ourselves, we're sparing them a slow, gruesome death by the claw and jaw of the carnivore.*
- *Nature is brutal and cruel. At least humans kill animals humanely.*
- *A knife to the throat or a bullet in the head is merciful compared to how these animals would die in the wild.*
- *We have to milk cows for the sake of their health and comfort.*
- *If we didn't breed animals, they wouldn't be here. We give animals life.*

- *If we stopped eating animals, entire industries would collapse and people would lose their jobs.*
- *If we stopped eating animals, they would go extinct. Is that what vegans want? I thought they cared about animals.*

Declarations like these—justifications we make to ourselves and one another—become the mantras that lull us into a trance of complacent consumption, even if that consumption means that we, ourselves, are harmed. In *Willful Blindness*, Heffernan illustrates this with what she calls "one of the most cognitively dissonant industries of the modern age: the tanning salon."[18] She tells us of people who regularly use tanning beds and refuse to believe the harm they cause—even when the research is staring them right in the face, even when they themselves develop skin cancer. Surely, they argue, tanning salons wouldn't be legal if they were harmful—right? "The very fact that they are viable, profitable businesses and that they are regulated is taken as proof that they must be safe—because otherwise they would be prohibited. That is as powerful a form of social validation as it is possible to find," Heffernan explains. She quotes a dermatologist who sees evidence of this willful blindness on a regular basis: "You get the most extraordinary vehemence from people who've been using the sun beds constantly. They're prepared to shout at me, insisting they are not harmful. There was one lady, we'd been quite friendly. She said, 'I use sun beds all the time and I love it and you aren't going to stop me. I don't want to know.' What's so sad about these patients is that they do know tanning is bad for you—that's why they're embarrassed—but they choose not to know."

Unfortunately, this denial outlives its victims and holds sway over the public's perceptions. Although most people know that exposure to UV radiation can lead to (sometimes fatal) diseases—just as most people know the consumption of animal flesh and fluids can lead to (sometimes fatal) diseases—they don't stop. Just as the meat, dairy, and egg industries tout the health benefits of their products, so too does the tanning industry promote the health benefits of tanning. Despite the fact that the US Department of Health and Human Services defines tanning beds and sun lamps as "known carcinogens" and countless peer-reviewed studies implicate the consumption of animal products as one of the primary causes of chronic disease and death in the United States, millions of Americans partake on a daily basis. Why? Fear of change. Ingrained habits. The need to belong. And the messages we receive from everyone around us, including industries themselves.

## THE STORIES WE ARE TOLD

Just as we choose willful blindness rather than let ourselves be thrust into unknown territory, so too do the members of our social circle have a stake in having us remain asleep, willfully blind, and self-deluded. After all, if they encouraged or embraced our awakening, not only might it force them to look at their own self-delusion, it could potentially shatter the very foundation upon which their relationship with us is built. We choose like-minded friends with whom we can rationalize our behavior, and we stave off dissent with the tacit threat of ostracism—the worst possible punishment for creatures oriented toward conformity and social inclusivity the way humans are. The desire to feel included and validated by others reaps so many physiological, psychological, social, and emotional rewards that it can blind us to the negative consequences of our actions—especially if they're consequences we can't see or touch, such as the hardening of our arteries, the gruesomeness of slaughterhouses, or the prevalence of greenhouse gases. And so, we tell ourselves and each other what we need to in order to keep the boat from rocking—even if the stories we tell are lies. *The animals are treated humanely. Cows have to be milked or they would die. Fish don't feel pain.*

Ironically, in a way, it's our compassion that motivates these lies. It's precisely because my parents knew how painful it would have been for me to know that I was contributing to violence against animals that they conjured up stories of suicidal chickens and masochistic pigs ("Animals are here for us; they sacrifice themselves so we can eat."). They weren't trying to hurt me; they were trying to protect me. It was their sensitivity—and their awareness of mine—that compelled them to romanticize what is in truth a very ugly endeavor, and millions of parents around the world do the same with their own children. The very idea that animals suffer because of our actions is so anathema to us—so difficult to confront—that instead of doing so, we idealize our use and abuse of them to the point of fantasy.

> The very idea that animals suffer because of our actions is so difficult to confront that instead of doing so, we idealize our use and abuse of them to the point of fantasy.

We do it as individuals, we do it as group members, and we do it as customers of the companies we pay billions of dollars to churn out tons of animal flesh and fluids each year. In turn, they spend millions of those same dollars marketing back to us the story we want to tell and be told. The genius of the animal exploitation industries lies in their awareness of our compassion and desire for optimal health, as well as our need to remain willfully blind to animal suffering. They *know* we feel terrible eating the animals they kill for us. They *know* we want to perceive ourselves as making compassionate, healthful choices. So in order to alleviate our discomfort and guilt, they propagandize the tale that animals gleefully give their lives for our pleasure and that meat, dairy, and eggs are health-promoting foods. The story we pay them to tell us is that animals are happy, willing, and eager to die on our behalf, that "milk does a body good," or that "eggs are nature's perfect food." It's a win-win: the companies sell us bits and pieces of animals (whom we have neither the stomach nor the heart to dismember ourselves), and their marketing campaigns enable us to enjoy the comfort of perceiving ourselves as compassionate and health-seeking people without the inconvenience of having to change our habits.

Several years ago, I spent a lot of time on a blog called *Suicide Food* that was created to be a clearinghouse of advertising images that depict "animals who act as though they wish to be consumed." Sadly but not surprisingly, the blog founders had no trouble compiling hundreds of images of ostensibly masochistic, cannibalistic, and suicidal animals—everyone from pigs, goats, cows, chickens, ostriches, and turkeys to shrimps, fishes, octopuses, crabs, frogs, and worms. Sexualized, feminized, and vying to be killed and consumed, some of them even participate in their own dismemberment—while alive, conscious, and smiling. Even without the invaluable contribution of the *Suicide Food* blog, I have my own vivid memories of "suicidal animals," the most famous of whom being Charlie the Tuna. Created in 1961 (and recently revived), this hipster mascot of the StarKist tuna company was single-minded in pursuit of his ostensible goal: to be impaled on a hook, killed, processed, canned, and eaten. But try as he might to be caught, the hook always eluded him—his disappointment answered with a disingenuous apology: "Sorry, Charlie." The creator of Suicide Food observed: "A fish goes to great lengths to connive, to trick, to persuade The Man to kill him. He grabs for the hook, only to see it snatched away again and again. And again. And again. We are meant to pity him. And we do."[19] And to demonstrate how much we pity him, we eat him. Again. And again. And again. His conscious demise is our guiltless pleasure. And so, it follows, out of similarly delusional self-perceived altruism, we breed, confine, manipulate, mutilate, and kill billions of animals a year—and drive many animals, such as the case with some species of tuna, to the brink of extinction.

For decades, corporations have used such tactics—from anthropomorphizing and cute-ifying animals to using images of animals to sell related products (for example, using a depiction of a pig to sell bacon)—in the process contributing to the public's collective willful ignorance regarding animal suffering and exploitation. Whether it's the "Eat Mor

Chikin" campaign by Chick-fil-A (featuring "activist cows" who promote the consumption of chickens—actually making the cows complicit in chickens' deaths) or the California Milk Advisory Board's "Happy Cow" ad campaigns ("Great milk comes from Happy Cows. Happy Cows come from California"), the result is a widening of the gap between our affection for animals and our hunger to consume their flesh and fluids.

Another way these industries encourage us to stay willfully blind is through the euphemistic language they use to talk about the violence they inflict on animals as well as to characterize the nutritional components of meat, dairy, and eggs. From the Greek word *euphmismos*, meaning "auspicious speech," euphemisms have their place in our interactions with others—to soften the blow of bad news, to comfort a grieving friend, or to avoid deliberately hurting someone's feelings. In such situations, euphemisms are a kindness. They help prevent pain and make the unpleasant more palatable. It's problematic, however, when euphemistic words disguise the truth and make the unacceptable acceptable. Examples of terms that mask our discomfort with and guilt about our use and abuse of nonhuman animals abound: Animals are "crops" and "stocks" who are "processed" in "packing plants." Hunters pursue "game," "dress" animals they've killed, and display their heads as "trophies." The government "culls" and "depopulates" large groups of individuals. Cows don't lactate; they "give milk." And so on.

The meat, dairy, and egg industries go to great lengths to remove words that would offend us and replace them with less emotive or provocative language. This is evident not only in their carefully chosen public-facing labeling terms and marketing lingo, but also in their internal literature, training manuals, and workplace terminology. Avoiding the more accurate but graphic term "beak burning," the egg and poultry industries instead refer to the standard industry practice of burning or cutting off the tips of birds' beaks without anesthesia as "beak conditioning," "beak trimming," and "beak treatment."[20] Instead of "toe burning" or "toe mutilation," the standard industry practice of cutting or burning off the tips of birds' toes without anesthesia, the poultry industries euphemistically call it "toe clipping" or "toe conditioning." Rather than saying an animal has been "bled to death," the preferred industry term is "exsanguinated."

The egg industry uses "hen rejuvenation" rather than "forced molting" to refer to the common practice of artificially inducing molting in hens, which tricks hens' already-stressed bodies into another egg-laying cycle by exposing them to constant light for seven days at a time. The pork industry disapproves of the use of "gestation crates" and "farrowing crates" to refer to the constrictive pens they confine pregnant pigs in and instead refers to them by the innocuous-sounding "maternity pens" or the Orwellian "individual gestation accommodations." Both the pig and veal industries avoid referring to these instruments of confinement as "crates," using "cribs" or "stalls" instead. When referring to the accepted industry practice of killing "nonviable piglets" by slamming their heads against floors or walls, they call it "manually applied blunt force trauma." Internally within the industry, it's known simply as "Ma-BFT"[21] or "thumping."

Industry terms once found only in trade journals have become commonplace in the public's vernacular. Rather than talking about animals being "killed" or "slaughtered," we use such terms as "harvested" and "processed," evoking pleasant thoughts of carrots being pulled from the ground or fruit being blended into a smoothie instead of the difficult and bloody act of slitting an animal's throat with a blade. Such euphemistic jargon is displayed unabashedly in industry press releases, marketing materials, and industry-supported legislation, setting an example for the public to follow. And we do follow, all the while staying blissfully ignorant and willfully unaware, trusting that the industries are well regulated, that they adhere to welfare standards, and that when they don't it's the exception rather than the rule—that it's just a few "bad apples."

The animal agriculture industry and the politicians who rely on its deep pockets know that words matter, which is why they work so hard to conceal the reality of their practices and products from the public—linguistically and literally, even going so far as to make it a crime to document their own practices. Euphemistically called "Agricultural Security Acts" or "Commerce Protection Acts" by the animal exploitation industries and the legislators who support them, ag-gag laws (a term coined by food writer Mark Bittman) started appearing a couple of decades ago to silence whistleblowers, journalists, undercover investigators, and the general public from revealing abuses in the animal agriculture industry. These ag-gag laws conceal animal cruelty by making it difficult to document animal agriculture practices via undercover or direct methods on ranches, in animal factories, on animal farms, and in slaughterhouses.

Ag-gag laws currently exist in six states—Alabama, Arkansas, Iowa, Kansas, Missouri, and North Carolina. After declaring them unconstitutional violations of the First Amendment, federal judges struck down ag-gag laws in Idaho and Utah, but lawmakers friendly to the animal agriculture industry have proposed such bills in numerous states and will continue to do so as long as they think they can get away with it. When these bills fail (and nearly all have), it's because constituents oppose them in the name of free speech and free press, but ironically, many of these constituents—who most likely oppose animal abuse—are often the same people who avoid looking at the undercover footage of animal farms and factories in the first place. If we genuinely honor truth and transparency, the least we can do is look, listen, and learn about the grim realities of the industries that bring animals into this world only to use, abuse, and kill them for profit—profit made at the expense of animals and on the reliability of our willful ignorance.

> The least we can do is look, listen, and learn about the grim realities of the industries that bring animals into this world only to use, abuse, and kill them for profit.

When the animal exploitation industries fail on the legislative front, they focus their efforts on the consumer sector, working to hinder the success of cruelty-free competitors. Despite already having the advantage of government subsidies and buybacks and the ears of the politicians they lobby, meat, dairy, and egg companies around the world are trying (and in some cases succeeding) to ban the words "meat," "milk," "yogurt," "butter," "ice cream," and other descriptors from the names of plant-based versions. If there's no animal source, they argue, then companies shouldn't be allowed to use such words to describe their products, even if they include such qualifiers as "vegan," "vegetarian," or "plant-based." Their goal is to make it illegal for companies to call their products "almond *milk*," "veggie *burger*," "soy *hot dog*," or "coconut *ice cream*," for instance, dubiously claiming that these words confuse and dupe consumers who think they are buying animal products. Of course this is subterfuge at its finest. If they were really so concerned about consumers not being duped, they wouldn't use euphemistic doublespeak to refer to their own abusive practices. If they really valued candor and openness, they wouldn't try to make it illegal to expose animal and environmental abuses.

## THE TRUTH WE DEFLECT

Whether they're trying to change laws or language, the meat, dairy, and egg companies employ these tactics to obscure the truth and keep the public willfully blind. But as individuals who don't want to wake up—or, to continue the blindness metaphor, *regain our sight*—we do the same thing. We may not support *criminalizing* the truth or making felons of those who expose it, but we certainly *demonize* those who do, such as when a vegan shows up, acting as a physical reminder of everything we work so hard to forget. As I explained earlier in this chapter, most of us consciously choose willful blindness in order to cope with the dissonance we feel participating in behaviors that are antithetical to our values. We go to great lengths to avoid conflict and guilt by trying to will the source of our conflict out of existence (*out of sight, out of mind*). But then a vegan shows up and smashes our illusion—ruining all our meat, dairy, and egg-eating fun.

The vegan doesn't have to actively proselytize; she just has to exist. As a result, nonvegans may recoil, retreat, defend, and deflect—anything to avoid the dissonance. And this may happen before a vegan even opens her mouth. Her very presence is an affront. *Don't tell me about how animals suffer; I don't want to know. Don't show me what animals endure; I don't want to look. Don't tell me how unhealthy this burger is; I want to enjoy it.* So, out of allegiance to our collective blissful ignorance and with the hope of resolving our dissonance, rather than condemn the abuses, we condemn the vegan.

- *Vegans are so holier-than-thou. They think they're better than everyone else.*
- *Vegans care more about animals than people.*
- *Vegans are in denial about how the food chain works. Animals eat other animals. That's life.*
- *Vegans are sick and unwell. They're deprived of nutrition that comes only from animal products.*
- *Vegans are extreme.*
- *Vegans are overly sentimental.*
- *Vegans are neurotic.*
- *Vegans have food issues. Vegans are overweight/underweight.*

And conveniently, with all this talk of vegans, no one is talking about the animals. Or the peer-reviewed studies that confirm the health ramifications that come from eating them. Or the environmental degradation directly linked to the production of meat, dairy, and eggs. The vegan becomes a handy diversion for the willfully blind. "It's like fingers pointing at the moon," as the traditional Buddhist metaphor goes. "If you watch the finger, you can't see the moon." In other words, in service of retaining that blindness, we attribute the ugliness not to the truth, which would compel us to change, but to those who reveal the truth.

Several years ago, I received a letter from a young woman who did a report for school about pigs. As a result, she stopped eating pigs. Time went by, and she did another report, this time about chickens, and she stopped eating chickens. Soon after, she did a report about cows and stopped eating cows. Her mother told her to stop doing reports. She knew that the more her daughter learned, the more she would wake up—the more her behavior would change. *Don't stop killing animals! Stop writing reports about killing animals! That's the problem: reports!* Shoot the messenger and hinder the truth. Censure the vegan and undermine what she represents. The only problem is it doesn't work. It may buy us a little more sleep, but try as we might, our pesky conscience just won't stay dormant. Like a slow intravenous drip, little by little, things start to stir, and the sleeper begins to awaken. That is the power and persistence of truth.

Despite every excuse we make and every myth we perpetuate; despite social pressure, expensive marketing campaigns, euphemistic language meant to blind us, laws meant to keep abuses hidden; and despite our own efforts to stay asleep, still we wake up. Despite an array of forces compelling us to remain blissfully ignorant, still millions of people become informed. Through some kind of encounter—a book they read, a pamphlet they're given, a documentary they watch, an animal they interact with, a vegan they meet—they experience what can only be described as an epiphany: a sudden revelation that compels them to align their behavior with their values, to make the dissonance consonant, to *become* vegetarian or vegan. In other words, to fully manifest the compassion that has always been inside of them, to choose life and wellness over sickness and death. To become awake.

The irony is that the very thing we were most afraid of—looking at the reality behind our consumption of animals—is the very thing that liberates us. We realize that the peace of mind we hoped to get from choosing *blissful ignorance* will elude us until we choose *disquieting awareness*, and the only way to get there is by bearing witness—by opening our eyes and being willing to look. We make ourselves powerless when we turn away from reality; only when we have all the information and are informed citizens do we have the power to do something. If we don't look, not only do we shirk our own responsibility, we also abdicate our power and deny the best of ourselves. As Heffernan found in her research, "We may have thought that being blind would make us safer, when in fact it leaves us crippled, vulnerable, and powerless. But when we confront facts and fears, we achieve real power and unleash our capacity for change. We give

> The very thing we were most afraid of—looking at the reality behind our consumption of animals—is the very thing that liberates us.

ourselves hope when we insist on looking. The very fact that willful blindness is willed . . . is what gives us the capacity to change it."[22]

So what is it that causes us to wake up? What are the encounters that lead to an epiphany? What compels some people to choose awareness over ignorance? That's what we'll explore in the next chapter.

### Chapter Two

# The Awakening

## *The Epiphany That Changes Everything*

> At the same moment, the hour of disenchantment
> having come, the princess awoke.
> —Charles Perrault, *The Sleeping Beauty in the Wood*

*Sleep/loss of consciousness* is a common archetype in many of the fairy tales that have permeated our literature for hundreds of years, as is its counterpart: *wakefulness/awareness*. In contemporary versions of *Sleeping Beauty* and *Snow White* as well as in similar stories throughout the world (*Brunhilde, Little Briar Rose, The Maiden with the Rose on Her Forehead*), the titular main characters are lulled to sleep by some kind of irresistible influence until they are finally awakened by a power greater than the original spell.

As we have seen—through the process of desensitization, willful blindness, and cognitive dissonance—the unconditional compassion we feel as children toward living animals gets put to sleep in favor of the pleasure and convenience of eating their flesh and fluids. But despite the social, institutional, and political mechanisms conspiring to keep us asleep, cracks begin to appear, often leading to some kind of encounter that forces us to confront what we had long been avoiding: the truth. Many vegans (and vegetarians) describe this experience as a kind of awakening—as if being revived from a trance or a spell. It's the wake-up call we'd been ignoring for years. Many describe it as an epiphany. Etymologically speaking, *epiphany* comes from a Greek word meaning "to come suddenly into view"—a perfect characterization of the moment when our deepest values are manifested right before our very eyes. The world remains the same, but the lens through which we see the world is completely altered.

> Despite the social, institutional, and political mechanisms conspiring to keep us asleep, cracks begin to appear, forcing us to confront what we had long been avoiding.

I've received thousands of letters over the years I've been helping people through this journey, and a similar vocabulary runs through all of the stories—a lexicon of *awakening*: words and phrases that speak to the disillusionment that comes with awareness:

"I had been oblivious."

"It's like I had been sleepwalking."

"It's as if I had been in a trance."

"I had been turning a blind eye."

"And then it clicked."

"The penny dropped."

"A light went on."

"A switch was flipped."

"The blinders were removed."

"A veil was lifted."

"I felt reborn."

"I've woken up."

*I once was lost, but now am found*
*Was blind but now I see.*

The trigger for this wake-up call is different for everyone. It can be emotional or cognitive, physical or spiritual, a deliberate journey or an unexpected surprise, but ultimately something happens that challenges our beliefs, shifts our perceptions, and compels us to change our behavior. Something clicks that leads us to ask new questions, to follow a different path, to nourish seeds that had been planted many years prior to this moment. We may not even know what we're looking for on this quest; we just know we need something different. We know that what worked before isn't quite working for us now, and our search leads to some kind of encounter. *When the student is ready, the teacher appears*, as the saying goes, and the teacher in our case can appear in many guises—in a person or an animal, a podcast or a book, a video or a photo. Sometimes all it takes is a few words—someone saying something in a way that yanks our head out of the sand. And it's at this moment—through this encounter—that we have our epiphany.

In our fairy tale motif, it's when the princess wakes up and the spell is broken. In our reality, the awakening might be an overt health crisis or the natural progression of a spiritual journey. It might be the death of a loved one (including a companion animal) or an encounter with a living animal that reminds us of the sentience of *all* animals. It might be new information we stumble upon that compels us to do more research. Whatever it is, it pushes us off the fence—a fence we may not have even known we were teetering on—and we land on the other side. Although the specific triggers that compel someone to wake up—to become vegan—are unique to each of us, and although there are always exceptions, I've found that these epiphanies can be broken down into distinct categories.

For some people, an epiphany occurs when they see farmed animals in person or in a video and realize there is no difference between them and the dogs and cats they know and love.

"I saw a YouTube video of a little girl playing an accordion alongside a field. A herd of cattle came running up to her and peacefully formed an audience, clearly curious and delighted. I looked over at my dog, a rescued Great Dane who I often call 'Cow' because of her size and goofy demeanor and suddenly, the lightbulb went off. In that moment, I knew unquestioningly in my heart that we are all complex, intelligent beings who are more alike than different. I became a vegetarian that very moment, and within a week, I was vegan."

"The whispers of vegetarianism/veganism have always been present in my life, but I ignored them. That whisper turned into a murmur, to a voice, to a full-blown shout that I couldn't ignore anymore. It happened while eating a chicken sandwich and watching my beloved birds eating at my bird feeder. If I wasn't willing to eat *them*, why was I willing to eat other animals? I thought I was living a compassionate lifestyle but now saw a glaring disconnection with my ideals. I finally listened and woke up."

"One day, I came across a photo online of a beautiful cat with the caption 'RIP' underneath. I didn't even know who this cat was, but my eyes filled with tears immediately, and all the feelings I had stopped myself from feeling rushed out. How could I feel so much for this dead cat but eat the bodies of other animals who valued their lives just as much? How could I continue to have blood on my hands? I quit eating animal products that moment and have never looked back."

"As part of my journey, I decided to visit a farm animal sanctuary. Once I looked these beautiful, gentle, kind creatures in the eyes I knew there was no going back for me. I was vegan for life."

"I was walking my dog, who made friends with a calf, and I realized there is no difference between that cow and my dog. I became vegetarian that day, and my journey continued from there. Once my heart was open, there was no going back."

For others, it's a health scare, accident, or other crisis that sets them on a new path.

"After being diagnosed with stage-three breast cancer last fall, I embarked on a journey to get well. Included in that journey was the realization that I had to make nutrition and lifestyle changes. I started researching and listening to your podcast, and I couldn't get enough of the information I was learning. Not only did I now have the knowledge I needed to improve my nutrition, I had a true motivation and inspiration to stay with it and make it a permanent lifestyle change."

"Being diagnosed with HIV was terrifying, but it was also one of the best things that could have happened to me. I was wasting my life working two jobs, going home and watching Netflix, eating junk food constantly, and smoking a pack of cigarettes a day. HIV made me realize that I've got only one life, and I shouldn't be living it that way. Almost a year later, I finally decided to become healthier. I was going to the gym and trying to eat better, then I met my online vegan friend and he helped me get the information I needed to make the change to a vegan lifestyle. I found your *30-Day Vegan Challenge* book and your *Food for Thought* podcast and I was hooked."

"A few years ago, I broke both my legs in a rock-climbing accident, had to undergo several surgeries, and was temporarily confined to a wheelchair. During rehabilitation I had a lot of time to read and think about my life. I stumbled upon a book that challenged my belief that 'going vegan' was extreme and that I would never be able to do it. As I became drawn into the arguments and then found your podcast, I started making connections and could no longer live with the knowledge about how cruelly animals are treated; how our health and environment suffer from consuming animal products; and how our human values lack humanity. I became vegan."

"I have to admit, after a diagnosis of celiac and having severe stomach pain for the past few months, my original reason for trying a plant-based diet was to ease all of that pain. However, after a few days in, I watched a number of documentaries and was absolutely horrified and disgusted about the way animals are being exploited. After this week and a half of eating plant-based and feeling so incredible, I can honestly say I am never going back to eating animals and their secretions. I have never felt more connected to myself, the earth, and my morals than I do now."

"In the beginning my concerns were more about my own health and the environment than about the animals. I began following a 'vegan before six' diet, never thinking that I would one day go completely vegan. But as I learned more about all the terrible ways that we humans mistreat our fellow Earthlings, I completely lost any desire to eat animals or their secretions."

For many, they encounter new information (through videos, documentaries, books, podcasts, or pamphlets), which leads to new realizations.

"An undercover video shown on the news was what did it for me. Once I saw how much damage, pain, and death I had caused in my life by not thinking and not making the connection, I was horror-stricken, and I stopped eating animals that day."

"I sat myself down and watched a documentary about animal abuse. It took me three very traumatic days to get through it all, but by the end I was well and truly a vegan first and foremost for animals, and since then I haven't looked back."

"After I watched a documentary about animals, I became vegan overnight. I didn't want to live in denial anymore."

"For my entire life, I was an out-and-out supreme meat-eater. There had been underlying thoughts and realizations that raised their ugly heads over the years—especially because I considered myself a conscientious person—but I somehow managed to box them up. One day while watching an animal documentary, all the boxes burst at once, and it came time to face the truth and put my money where my mouth was. I became vegan."

"This time last year I watched your talk online about veganism and realized I couldn't continue participating in the suffering. I took a deep breath, opened my heart, put my faith in compassion, and became vegan."

Some people are led to veganism because they care about environmental and other social issues.

"I started learning about veganism last year while doing a presentation about feminism and somehow stumbled upon animal welfare. It really made me angry to see what is happening to both women and animals, and I couldn't ignore the parallels in the exploitation of both. I became vegan, and I've never looked back."

"I have always been passionate about the environment and animal welfare, but still led a carnivorous lifestyle. In a video I watched, someone made the point that you cannot say you're really concerned about the environment and still eat meat. That was what led me to become vegan."

"I am a student at Copenhagen University, where I am doing a masters in English and History. This semester I am doing a course on food and agriculture in Denmark from 1880 to 2010. As a result of my studies, I started thinking seriously about the environmental effects of meat consumption, and all my buried disgust with meat came to the surface once again. One day I was suddenly a vegetarian. It wasn't really a conscious decision, I just couldn't eat meat anymore. I started researching and reading more. I bought a couple of cookbooks and started listening to podcasts, and that was it. I became vegan. I honestly never thought I would be vegan, but I now see the world in a completely different way."

"I had always considered myself to be environmentally friendly, but the impact of the meat industry on our environment was completely unknown to me, and it was mind-blowing to learn about it. I stopped eating meat and continued from there."

"I would consider myself a strong advocate for social and environmental justice and having studied the dynamics of sexism, racism, classism, capitalism, etc., I have learned to connect the dots in most types of power relations and to see past the charade that maintains the status quo. In one of your podcast episodes, when you spoke about the systems that are set up to help make meat-eaters complacent, it really hit me. All of these other systems of power that I've been fighting against (even including food systems) are all connected, and I really can't continue to support industries that threaten so much that I value. Because it's all connected, in order to undo one type of oppression and injustice I need to undo all of them. I can no longer eat anything that comes from an animal."

"Not eating animals is consistent with the way I've already been living my life, consistent with my beliefs about nonviolence and human rights, about compassion and reducing suffering in the world. I can't believe it took me this long, but I'm so grateful that I finally 'got it.'"

Many who are already vegetarian—whether for health or ethical reasons—realize that becoming vegan is the next natural step in the continuum.

"I've been a vegetarian the majority of my life, without having any strong ethical convictions. As ignorant as it may sound, I pictured ol'

Bessie grazing on green pastures and getting milked from time to time throughout the day. Consuming dairy products and animal byproducts didn't cause me the pain that it does today because I just didn't know. Out of sight, out of mind. After watching fifteen minutes of a documentary, I just said, 'I'm done,' and indeed, that marked the beginning of my awakening."

"Vegetarian for many years, I was on the edge of becoming vegan, so when I listened to a few podcasts, I finally felt like I had no choice but to drop the dairy and eggs. It was such a wonderful day for me, and although I cried a lot over those coming weeks and months, it was very cathartic."

"I had been telling myself I was living guilt-free and not causing any harm to animals due to my vegetarianism. I had always wondered about milk, eggs, wool, etc., but because animals weren't killed for these things, I simply didn't second-guess any of it. I even judged vegans for being 'extreme.' After seeing a video clip online, I felt horrible. I immediately stopped eating any dairy or eggs and buying anything taken from an animal."

"There was a shadow in my heart that said being vegetarian wasn't enough. I didn't feel fully at peace until I became vegan after being open enough to learn more. I'm so grateful I did."

"I gave up red meat for ethical reasons early in high school, but I still ate fish and fowl for many years after. I've known about their suffering, and I blocked it from my mind so I could enjoy consuming their products in blissful ignorance. I don't know what changed in me. Maybe it was my realization that what I was eating wasn't doing my body any favors. Maybe it was an accumulation of sorrow for all of the lives lost in order to selfishly feed myself. But the consciousness shift came, and I became vegan."

"Having been vegetarian for ten years and never really thinking I needed to go vegan, after watching an animal documentary, my perception changed instantly."

I've also heard from a number of people whose epiphany arose out of empathy for the mother/baby bond experienced by all mammals.

"For me, it was breastfeeding my daughters and learning how dairy cows are treated. To know that another mother cannot be with and nurture her little one the way I am able to because they are taken from her breaks my heart."

"For some reason, I didn't realize that dairy cows have to be kept pregnant/have babies in order to produce milk. And I definitely never realized how many baby cows are taken abruptly from their mother and slaughtered so that I could eat my dairy. Once I found that out, giving up dairy and staying off dairy has not been a problem."

"I had never thought it through that cows didn't just 'give milk' without having a baby and that male babies were useless to the industry and thus disposed of."

"It was gut-wrenching to learn about what happens to male chicks in the egg industry and baby cows in the dairy industry. I never knew that dairy cows have to be pregnant full-time to give milk. It's basic biology, I know, but somehow I overlooked it."

"In a documentary I watched, there's a scene of a mother cow being separated from her baby and there's also a story of chickens who were rescued and walk on the ground for the first time. On our way home from watching the film, I said to my husband, 'I don't ever again want to contribute to that kind of suffering,' and he replied, 'I'm with you.' We went home and threw out everything in our kitchen that wasn't vegan and have been vegan ever since that day."

"For me, when I learned that calves are torn away from their mothers, that was it. I never really thought about how we get our milk, but when I learned this piece of information, that was all I needed!"

"I was a vegetarian for about eight years, for animals mostly. While I was on holiday, I visited a dairy farm, where they sold ice cream made with their dairy. You could see most of the farm, including the milking robot and stables where the cows were. Two very young calves were somewhere else in another part of the farm, separated from their moms. I could see the umbilical cords. They were so desperate for a cuddle and were trying to suckle on everything, mostly visitors' hands. That was it for me; I wanted no part of this."

"I grew up surrounded by dairy farms, took class trips to them and had no idea cows didn't 'give milk.' Learning they are mammals (duh!), and only produce milk because they were forced to have a calf, did it. I felt lied to, tricked, duped, and stupid that I didn't know that for twenty-eight years of my life."

What is so striking in story after story is how adept we are at not seeing what's right in front of us—so much so that even those who work in the animal exploitation industries are capable of inuring themselves to the suffering animals endure and of denying their part in the slaughter process. They battle the same dissonance we all do—but it's multiplied tenfold in the name of their livelihood, their family business, or their very identity. Many ranchers talk about intentionally never ascribing a personality to or having a relationship with their animals so as not to become emotionally attached to them. Very few name their animals for the same reason. Unbelievable as it sounds, I've heard from people who grew up on dairy farms but who never realized that cows had to be pregnant in order to lactate, that calves were taken away from their mothers, or that the adult cows were sent to slaughter after only a few years. Many farmers and ranchers will admit to never accompanying

> What is so striking in each epiphany story is how adept we are at not seeing what's right in front of us.

their animals to the slaughterhouse because they don't want to see how they end up. And many slaughterhouses are designed to keep the majority of the workers blind to—and thus guiltless in—the actual killing.

In his book *Every Twelve Seconds: Industrialized Slaughter and the Politics of Sight*, Timothy Pachirat describes how slaughterhouses are divided into separate departments or "zones of confinement" that shield most of the workers from the actual killing and thus the complicity associated with this type of work:

> Of 121 distinct "kill floor jobs" that I map and describe in the book, only the "knocker" both sees the cattle while sentient and delivers the blow that is supposed to render them insensible. The knocker is the worker who stands at the knocking box and shoots each individual animal in the head with a captive bolt steel gun. On an average day, this lone worker shoots 2,500 individual animals at a rate of one every twelve seconds.
>
> There is a kind of collective mythology built up around this particular worker, a mythology that allows for an implicit moral exchange in which the knocker alone performs the work of killing, while the work of the other 800 slaughterhouse workers is morally unrelated to that killing. It is a fiction, but a convincing one: of all the workers in the

slaughterhouse, only the knocker delivers the blow that begins the irreversible process of transforming the live creatures into dead ones. If you listen carefully enough to the hundreds of workers performing the 120 other jobs on the kill floor, this might be the refrain you hear: "Only the knocker." It is simple moral math: the kill floor operates with 120 + 1 jobs. And as long as the 1 exists, as long as there is some plausible narrative that concentrates the heaviest weight of the dirtiest work on this 1, then the other 120 kill floor workers can say, and believe it, "I'm not going to take part in this."[1]

Even built into the slaughterhouse design itself is a literal and linguistic distancing that serves to reduce living, feeling, breathing beings to inanimate flesh. "From the moment cattle are unloaded from transport trucks into the slaughterhouse's holding pens," Pachirat explains, "managers and kill floor supervisors refer to them as 'beef.'" The physical barriers, the rigid divisions of labor, and the use of euphemistic language all have the seductive effect of concealing even slaughterhouse workers from reality. Pachirat opens the book with the story of a cow who escapes from a slaughterhouse near the one Pachirat was working in. After a long pursuit, the police corner the cow and shoot her dead in an alleyway. A number of workers who happened to be outside on break and witnessed the shooting expressed their anger, shock, and horror at the killing of this animal at the hands of the police. And yet, "at the end of lunch break, workers returned to work on a kill floor that killed 2,500 animals each day."[2]

> We are masters of willful blindness, and yet the potential for awakening is in us all.

We are indeed masters of willful blindness, and yet the potential for awakening is in us all. Those who work in the animal agriculture industry may—by necessity—have to quell their dissonance and discomfort more than most of us, but they're certainly not immune to having their own epiphany. Some become vegetarian and try to continue farming animals, but they soon discover that once the cracks start appearing, it's nearly impossible to close them up.

"We stood at the gate listening to one of our baby goats being driven away [to slaughter], crying in the trunk of the car. It was at this horrific moment when we looked at each other with tears in our eyes. We have since left the dairy industry and converted our farm into a sanctuary."[3]

—Cheri Ezell, former goat farmer

"One day, it was time to send one of the cows to the slaughterhouse and I decided to accompany him. I remember the car ride there so vividly, and then our arrival at the local 'humane slaughter' facility . . . there were rows of gentle animals standing there quietly. I remember being told 'the first time here is unpleasant for everybody.' I didn't stay to witness our steer being killed; we just dropped him off and I took a look around. But it was very difficult to leave him there. He was obviously disoriented and didn't want to go into his stall, so they had to force him in there . . . which happens pretty often. There was a large room filled with goats, sheep, and alpacas, and they were all just standing there quietly, nervously looking at me. They were scared and disoriented. It really seemed like they knew what was going on. It was horrifying to see so many babies in one room, waiting for their death. I never went to the slaughterhouse again, but that day really strengthened my resolve to help animals, and I became a passionate vegan."[4]

—Edith Barabash, former cattle ranch worker

"I spent forty-five years in the cattle business, always professing that I loved my animals. But it was years before I was willing to admit I was more interested in profit than the animals' health. The fact of it is, we simply raised them to a point where they became economically beneficial to us to sell. I finally woke up. Looking in those big old brown eyes, I realized those animals loved life in their way just as much as I loved life in mine; there was no way in the world I could ever put them to death again."[5]

        —Howard Lyman, former beef cattle rancher

"It's amazing what you can block out when you really put yourself into it. I, who had ten years earlier been reduced to tears watching under-cover videos of how farmed animals were treated on industrial farms, was now working on a 'humane' dairy farm where tiny newborn goats were taken away from their mothers immediately, their cries of distress ignored. I didn't think about it much. Several years later, my partner fell deeply in love with [a rescue Chihuahua named Dingo]. She texted me from work one day and said 'I'm going to need to become a vegan. I can't eat animals or animal products anymore.' The wall I'd built must have been very shoddy indeed because that was really all it took for me. We both became vegan that day and started a new path forward."[6]

        —Susana Romatz, former goat dairy farmer

"There was a bad accident just up from our job site. I was running a machine that day, had the heat cranked and was still bundled up. The traffic had come to a complete stop. I looked beside me on the highway and there was a tractor trailer hauling pigs to Quebec. That was the day I made the connection. I looked these poor animals in the eyes and I knew they were being sent to their deaths. It was now −36 and they were freezing! Their skin was red and you could see ice on some of their faces. My heart sank. I felt so bad for them and I told myself that was it! I will never cause harm to another creature again! I never looked back. After that, I never once thought if it would be hard to be a vegan and to give up all the meats and cheeses. My wife, daughter, and I are vegan for life! We also have three dogs and they consume a plant-based diet as well."[7]

        —Chris Mills, former hunter, trapper, and dairy farm worker

"The sense of horror was immediate. I saw mothers who had birthed in snow or storms have their babies taken immediately—they didn't even get to clean them first. The tiniest calves are tube-fed twice a day for four days, a liter of colostrum poured in all at once. I knew, logically, that cows need babies to produce milk, but I didn't really think about the fact those babies are almost immediately taken away from their mothers. That first morning, I knew I would never have dairy again and I cried every day for two weeks."[8]

—Jess Strathdee, former dairy farmer

Feelings of sadness, shock, and grief run through many people's stories of transformation, whether or not they've raised animals for slaughter, but these feelings are also mingled with a great sense of relief. Of catharsis. Of liberation. Of joy. Of wellness. The benefits new vegans experience—whether they're physical, emotional, mental, or spiritual—range from reversing heart disease, getting off medications, healing ailments, having more energy, and improving athletic performance to deepening their spiritual practice, connecting more with their values, experiencing an unexpected affection for animals, and feeling a sense of peace and purpose. In our fairy tale archetype, the story ends once the hero or heroine is awakened and goes on to "live happily ever after," but for us, our awakening is really just the beginning. Although there are many rewards—both tangible and intangible—the path of wakefulness is also fraught with obstacles and obstructions that can hinder our progress forward and make us lose our way—however pure our intentions and strong our will.

> Just as *becoming* vegan is a process, *being* vegan is a process as well. The secret to *staying* vegan is to realize that it, too, is a journey more than it is a destination.

One of the mistakes vegans tend to make is to think that once they've made the switch from nonvegan to vegan—once they've become awake—they've reached their goal and the journey is over. That they'll live happily ever after like our prototypal princess. The risk of such complacency is stagnancy, frustration, and powerlessness—which can result in giving up entirely and returning to the blissful state of willful blindness. Just as *becoming* vegan is a process, *being* vegan is a process as well. The secret to *staying* vegan is to realize that it, too, is a journey more than it is a destination.

*Section Two*

# STAYING VEGAN

n the decades I've been guiding people through the process of becoming and staying vegan, I've learned that the food is the easy part: people learn the practical aspects—what to eat, where to shop, how to cook—with considerable ease. More challenging is dealing with the social, cultural, and emotional aspects: being asked to defend yourself all the time, living with the acute awareness of animal suffering, people expecting you to have all the answers related to nutrition, anthropology, animal husbandry, ecology, and the culinary arts.

Add to that the unexpected resistance from friends, family members, and society at large, many of whom justify the consumption of meat, dairy, and eggs from a cultural, historical, social, evolutionary, and physiological perspective, and newly awakened vegans can wind up feeling isolated, uncertain, and disempowered. Feeling pressure to conform to the status quo, social norms, family expectations, and cultural mores, vegans can often feel they don't fit in anywhere. What's more, many burden themselves with unrealistic goals of perfection and purity, feeling guilty for having once eaten animals and shame for not stopping sooner. They see animal suffering wherever they turn and feel powerless to stop it, and they often avoid asking for their veganism to be accommodated lest they be viewed as high-maintenance or demanding.

No doubt this constant pressure takes its toll. No doubt this is why so many people give up and revert to eating animal flesh and fluids. No doubt this is why many who manage to remain vegan shy away from speaking out and coming out of the "vegan closet" or end up feeling angry, isolated, and misunderstood. As a result of being awake, despite making what initially feels like a positive change with many benefits and rewards, many vegans struggle socially and emotionally—and more often than not return to eating meat, dairy, and eggs.

In 2014, Faunalytics, a nonprofit organization that conducts essential research to help animal advocates increase their impact, partnered with Harris Interactive to survey the eating habits of 11,399 adults ages seventeen and older in order to examine "potential factors in people's decisions to either adopt or give up a vegetarian or vegan diet."[1] According to the findings of this "Study of Current and Former Vegetarians and Vegans," of those men and women who had at one time identified as being vegetarian or vegan, about 84 percent of them said they reverted to eating animals—despite having originally stopped out of genuine concern about animals, their health, or the environment. So, while millions of people have the desire to *become* vegan, what they lack are the tools and skills they need to *stay* vegan.

After hearing from thousands of people over the years who've become vegan, stopped being vegan, or struggled with staying vegan, I began to see common threads within all of their stories—threads that provide insight into why some people stay vegan and others don't, and threads that give name to the shared social experiences and challenges of everyone who stops eating meat, dairy, and eggs, whether they do so for health or ethical reasons. This next section summarizes each of these common experiences in the form of ten stages of being vegan, and lays out the practical skills needed to move through each of them productively and joyfully, with the hope of reducing the risk of returning to eating meat, dairy, and eggs. These stages provide validation for our present experience and act as signposts for what lies ahead, helping us avoid collisions and confusion.

My intention in presenting these ten stages is:

◆ to normalize this compassionate and healthful way of living
◆ to provide validation that what you experience is real and commonplace
◆ to cement veganism as a legitimate and pleasurable way of living and eating

- to offer assurance that you're not alone
- to provide a blueprint for you to sustain a life motivated by compassion and wellness
- to help you find comfort and clarity in your mind, your world, and your relationships

These stages position veganism not merely as an alternative to meat, dairy, and egg consumption, but as a valid ethic steeped in moral values and in the desire to thrive. These stages aren't linear (you can cycle through several in a day), and they certainly aren't mandatory (they're not stages to follow as much as they are experiences to identify with), but they reflect what most people experience once they make the transition, and they provide a guide to *staying* vegan—joyfully, proudly, and unwaveringly.

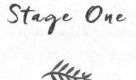

## Stage One

# Bearing Witness

## *Compassion Fatigue, Self-Care, and the Voracious Consumption of Information*

The mind, once stretched by a new idea, never
returns to its original dimensions.

—Ralph Waldo Emerson

Once awakened, sleep feels far away. Once you *know*, you can't *unknow*, and this stage is all about knowing and validating what we've come to know. By the time we get here, we've already had our epiphany. We've already had our awakening, but we're still adjusting to the light and rubbing the sleep out of our eyes. Fully awake and acutely aware, some of the first questions we ask ourselves are *How can this be real?* and *How can this be true?* It's not that we don't believe the facts that compelled us to become vegan, but we want to see with our own eyes. We want proof, evidence, corroboration, validation. We want documentation. This isn't a matter of the skeptic who needs to *see* in order to *believe*; it's more like we're making up for lost time and lost awareness, which produces an insatiable desire to consume everything we missed while we were sleeping. At this stage, we read every book we can get our hands on and watch every documentary. We seek out podcasts, videos, and websites. We drink in everything related to veganism, becoming intoxicated by the facts we avoided for so long. We watch animal slaughter videos with our mouths agape and our eyes filled with tears, determined to bear witness now that we're awake. We devour resources related to nutrition and health to confirm the benefits of a plant-based diet and to dispel any lingering notions that we're physiologically designed to thrive on animal flesh and fluids. We look for resources to confirm that we can transition our family healthfully or that we can still be strong and muscular, capable of competing in marathons and winning triathlons. We buy our first vegan cookbook and search the internet for recipes, excited to venture into a realm of new tastes and textures.

Like a newborn for whom the whole world is fresh, we feel vulnerable and curious, overwhelmed and passionate, bright-eyed and bushy-tailed. This is the point at which we begin sharing our newfound knowledge with everyone around us, prefacing most of our sentences with *Did you know . . . ?* or *I can't believe . . . !* or *I had no idea. . . .* We ask ourselves, *How can this be happening? This* might refer to the fact that nearly 70 billion land animals worldwide are brought into this world only to be killed (a conservative estimate considering the fact that some countries underreport).[1] *This* might refer to the fact that 1 to 3 trillion aquatic animals are killed each year by the global commercial fishing industry.[2] Or the fact that the majority of animals killed are not protected under any humane slaughter laws. Or the fact that those who are covered still experience immense pain and suffering. Or the fact that baby male chicks in the egg industry are killed upon hatching because they're useless in an industry that exploits the female reproductive system.

*This* might refer to the fact that animal agriculture is responsible for 14.5 percent of anthropogenic (human-caused) greenhouse gas emissions, more than the exhaust from all modes of transportation combined,[3] posing a fundamental threat to all life on this planet. *This* might refer to the fact that 2,500 gallons of water are needed to produce one pound of beef, 1,000 gallons of water for one gallon of cow's milk, 477 gallons for one pound of eggs, and 900 gallons for one pound of cheese.[4] Or that the US government kills millions of wild animals on public lands every year at the behest of private ranchers.[5]

Or that every minute, 7 million pounds of excrement are produced by animals raised for food in the US.[6] Or that for every pound of fish caught, up to five pounds of unintended marine species are caught and discarded as by-kill.[7] Or that animal agriculture is responsible for up to 91 percent of Amazon rainforest destruction.[8] Or that 80 percent of antibiotics sold in the United States are fed to livestock to keep animals healthy since the stressful conditions under which they're raised make them prone to disease.[9]

*This* might refer to the fact that there is a proven link between consumption of dairy products and autoimmune diseases.[10] Or that children suffer from ailments linked to dairy consumption.[11] Or that your chances of getting cancer if you eat meat are one in two if you're male and one in three if you're female.[12] Or to the fact that red meat intake is associated with an elevated risk of cardiovascular disease and cardiovascular death.[13]

Many of us on this journey may enter this first stage before we're fully vegan—when we're vegetarians or pescatarians. For instance, when I first stopped eating land animals after reading John Robbins's *Diet for a New America* but was still eating the flesh of aquatic animals and the milk and eggs of land animals, I wanted to know more about animal abuses and animal rights. Even though I was still half-asleep—I just didn't make the connection to the ethical and health considerations related to fish, cow's milk, and chicken's eggs—I read everything I could about other animal issues, including animal testing, puppy mills, circuses, and zoos, and decided then and there to become an advocate for animals. It took several years before I became fully awake—before I *became vegan*—but those early days of information-seeking laid the path for the journey that was still ahead of me.

In my quest to voraciously consume information, the first book I found (and one that I still have today) was called *Animal Rights: A Beginner's Guide—A Handbook of Issues, Organizations, Actions, and Resources* by Amy Blount Achor. I can still remember sitting in a library in New Jersey in 1992 carefully perusing that 420-page book, soaking up every word, poring over every photo, and feeling determined to do what I could to stop the atrocities. Several years later, I read *Slaughterhouse* by Gail Eisnitz, which knocked me into full consciousness, compelled me to *become vegan*, and inspired me to read every book I could find about animal protection and veganism. I devoured one book after another: *Animal Liberation* and *Ethics into Action: Henry Spira and the Animal Rights Movement* by Peter Singer, *The Case for Animal Rights* by Tom Regan, *An Unnatural Order* by Jim Mason, *The Dreaded Comparison* by Marjorie Spiegel, *Dead Meat* by Sue Coe, *Mad Cowboy* by Howard Lyman.

Even a couple of years after becoming vegan, I was still voraciously consuming information. I devoured every new animal rights book that came out, including *Rattling the Cage: Toward Legal Rights for Animals* by Steven M. Wise, *Eternal Treblinka: Our Treatment of Animals and the Holocaust* by Charles Patterson, and *Dominion: The Power of Man, the Suffering of Animals, and the Call to Mercy* by Matthew Scully. Consumed with questions and curious about nutrition, I was thrilled to find *Becoming Vegan* by Brenda Davis and Vesanto Melina; eager to cook delicious meals without animal products, I bought my first vegan cookbook: *The Peaceful Palate* by Jennifer Raymond. Full of simple recipes with recognizable ingredients, that cookbook became a mainstay for me and had a great influence on how I ate and cooked, especially in the beginning of my vegan journey. (The first books we read when we become vegan become such an intimate part of our story and a special part of our hearts, which is why I take it very seriously and am so moved when people tell me that my cookbooks were the first ones they ever bought.)

It was 1999 when I became vegan, and bookstores weren't exactly brimming with vegan and vegetarian cookbooks, but I managed to find a few others that are still in my collection, such as *Tofu Cookery* by Louise Hagler, *How It All Vegan* by Tanya Barnard and Sarah Kramer, and of course Joanne Stepaniak's classic, *Vegan Vittles*. Having been raised on typical, bland American cuisine, I had a limited palate when it came to flavors and seasonings, but becoming vegan broadened my options and expanded my tastes; as a result, my affinity for international cuisine increased, as did my variety of cookbooks. *The Enlightened Kitchen* by Mari Fujii was my first foray into traditional Japanese cuisine, *The Mediterranean Vegan Kitchen* and *Vegan Italiano* by Donna Klein helped me hone my Italian culinary skills, and Robin Robertson's *Vegan Planet* featured delicious recipes from around the world.

Podcasts were nonexistent then, but I do remember buying an audiotape of a keynote address by PETA president Ingrid Newkirk called "Speaking Up for Animals," and I must have listened to it a dozen times in the first several months I had it. When animal advocate and then-PETA staffer Bruce Friedrich made an audiotape called "Vegetarianism in a Nutshell" a couple years later, I listened until I had it memorized. At the time, there weren't a lot of documentary films available to watch, but I remember being thrilled to discover that *Diet for a New America* had been made into a documentary for public television—in 1991—and was able to find the VHS tape! (Yes, I realize I'm dating myself.) Ditto *A Cow at My Table*, which was a feature-length documentary film released the same year I went vegan. *Meet Your Meat*, a short film composed of scenes of animal slaughter from typical slaughterhouses, narrated by Alec Baldwin and produced by PETA, was not only something I watched a number of times, it was also the primary tool I used to help others bear witness. Tribe of Heart's film *The Witness,* which came out just a year after I went vegan, is the story of a builder turned animal advocate who rigs up his construction van with television screens to broadcast undercover footage of animals on fur farms. No doubt this film was the beginning of a new type of advocacy whereby undercover video footage is presented on screens in public places for passersby to watch and, in fact, it became one of my primary tools of advocacy after seeing this movie two decades ago (see Stage Nine: Finding Your Place). Inspired by other advocates doing the same, I started hosting my own "street TV" exhibits on public sidewalks in nearby towns. I bought a combination TV/VHS player, hit the streets, and screened a loop of *Meet Your Meat* every Friday night while handing out copies of the pamphlet *Why Vegan?* I watched people have their own epiphanies and heard them ask the same questions we all do once we know: *How can this be happening? How is this real?*

Prior to this point in our journey, many of us have already seen or heard something that compels us to change (like watching a video or seeing a news broadcast), but once we do—once we *become vegan*—we want to see more, we want to know more, and we can't stop staring. We feel we owe it to ourselves. We feel we owe it to the animals. And we do. It's for this reason that bearing witness, consuming information, and validating why we became vegan in the first place should *remain* part of our journey—even after we become vegan, and whether we become vegan for health or ethics.

> Once we *become vegan,* we want to see more, we want to know more, and we can't stop staring. We feel we owe it to ourselves. We feel we owe it to the animals. And we do.

To reiterate, none of these "stages" are mandatory. You don't *have to* voraciously consume information at this point, but it's very likely that you will feel compelled to. In fact, this is often when people who have become vegan for health reasons feel comfortable enough looking further into the ethics of veganism. No longer participating in the consumption of animals and thus relieved of any pangs of guilt, they often feel they have the mental and emotional capacity to learn more about what happens to animals—something they most likely avoided when they were still eating meat, dairy, and eggs. Similarly, people who become vegan for the animals initially tend to consume transitional foods such as vegan meats, cheeses, and eggs voraciously, almost as if making up for all the foods they thought they wouldn't be able to eat once they became vegan. Over time, however, they often begin learning more about the health benefits of incorporating more whole foods into their diet.

When it comes to witnessing what animals endure for our pleasure, profit, and palates, it's incredibly powerful, effective, and necessary to do so, but take heed: I'm not suggesting that we watch videos and read books to the point where we become despondent. I don't advocate masochism. I'm not saying we need to bear witness every day—or even every week. I'm also not saying that we should bear witness when we're already feeling low, hopeless, sad, or depressed. We need to pay attention to how we're feeling at the moment we choose to watch a video, look at a photo, or read an exposé of animal abuse, but I do believe that doing so now and again will remind us of what is so easily forgotten and so intentionally hidden from our sight. It also connects us with why we woke up in the first place.

Some people feel they don't need to be reminded about how bad things are—that once they go through their transformation it's unnecessary to ever have to look again. That may indeed be the case for some people, especially those of us who already have a supportive community and are surrounded by like-minded people who buttress our resolve. But, as I have said and will continue to emphasize: being vegan/being awake is a journey, not a destination. It's also not linear. We don't start at Stage One and end at Stage Ten with a certificate of completion. That's exactly the danger I would warn against; *there is no end point.* In other words, being awake doesn't mean you're immune from ever going back to sleep. You can absolutely fall asleep again, and that's why I recommend revisiting this stage—Bearing Witness—every so often. This will happen naturally if you're subscribed to mailing lists of vegan organizations, reading vegan blogs, or following animal advocates on social media, but even if you've read everything related to veganism and animal rights and have watched every documentary that's been made up to this point, don't ever stop. Read *more*. Watch *more*. Seek out *more* information. You may need to wait six months or a year before doing so, but never stop learning, never stop questioning. Whether you've been vegan for two years, five years, ten years, or more, never stop growing and challenging yourself—even if it stings a little. If we don't bear witness every so often, we risk forgetting. We risk losing our foundation, which could potentially lead us back to willful blindness.

> Being awake doesn't mean you're immune from ever going back to sleep. If we don't bear witness every so often, we risk forgetting.

How often you bear witness is up to you, but whenever you do, I highly recommend creating a plan in advance for coping with the distress of seeing graphic images or reading disturbing accounts of animal suffering. It can indeed be traumatic to see or hear about animals being tortured and killed, which is why most of us avoid it in the first place, so when exposing yourself to stories or images of animal exploitation and abuse, it's best to have a wellness plan in place first. Here are some suggestions for such a plan:

→ Watch a video or read a book along with someone you love and trust.
→ Have hankies close at hand.
→ Let yourself cry.

→ Let yourself feel whatever it is you're feeling—anger, despair, shock, sadness.

→ Spend a few minutes writing down your thoughts, feelings, and reactions *right after* you consume the information. Bearing witness can be painful, but it can also be cathartic and even constructive. You might wind up writing an op-ed or a letter to the editor based on what you've seen or read. You might write a post for your blog or social media feeds. You might decide to contact your legislators because of something you've learned. Use the time just after bearing witness to honor your feelings and also to express them in a constructive way.

I'd like to say that we always have agency in our lives to pick and choose what information we consume, but it's not uncommon to unwittingly come across an unsettling image or story while we're browsing the internet or for one to inadvertently pop up while we're scrolling through social media feeds. It can be jarring, to say the least. Create a plan for these occasions as well. Take a breath. Shed a tear. Scroll away. You can even hide the photo or unfollow the person who posted it. You're not betraying animals by being discerning about when and where you want to bear witness.

## AVOIDING BURNOUT

Some vegans feel they need to bear witness to the realities of animal abuse again and again and again as a testament to how much they care. But this is a sentiment (often an unconscious one) that borders on martyrdom—which is neither a sustainable nor a joyful way to live. While an enthusiastic desire to consume new information is a helpful and necessary part of this journey, voracious *overconsumption* of and prolonged exposure to distressing situations can create its own set of problems, namely a condition that has been called "compassion fatigue." First used to refer to the burnout that nurses, therapists, veterinarians, and others in health-care experience as they're exposed to protracted traumatic work scenarios, it's a term often used synonymously with post-traumatic stress disorder (PTSD) or secondary traumatic stress (STS). Characterized by a gradual lessening of compassion over time, compassion fatigue can happen to people who are trying to help those in distress. "It is an extreme state of tension and preoccupation with the suffering of those being helped," says Dr. Charles Figley of Tulane University, "to the degree that it can create a secondary traumatic stress for the helper."[14] Sufferers can exhibit a variety of symptoms including a sense of helplessness, powerlessness, guilt, or hopelessness; a decrease in experiences of pleasure; constant stress and anxiety; extreme sadness or depression; insomnia or nightmares; hyper-sensitivity; and a pervasive negative attitude. Those experiencing compas-sion fatigue tend to harbor anger, which leads to despair, which can lead to isolation, cynicism, substance abuse, and other forms of self-harm.

Truth be told, I don't like the term "compassion fatigue." I don't believe it is *compassion* that fatigues us, and I don't believe that we could ever have so much compassion that it would result in exhaustion, but I do believe that we can experience *empathic overarousal* or *empathic distress*, terms that are increasingly used by those who study burnout and that I think more accurately characterize exactly what is taking place. Empathy is important for understanding others' emotions, but feeling empathy can also be painful. "When we share the suffering of others too much, our negative emotions increase. It carries the danger of an emotional burn-out," says Olga Klimecki, a researcher who led and published a study that demonstrates how honing our own compassion skills results in a greater ability to cope with trauma and distress.[15]

In other words, *empathic distress is the problem. Compassion is the remedy.* The research team that conducted the study sent participants to a one-day loving-kindness meditation class as a way of cultivating their compassion skills and found that as a result, the study subjects were bet-ter able to experience "resilience and approach stressful situations with more positive affect." It's not that negative emotions disappeared after the loving-kindness training but that the participants were less likely to feel distressed themselves. "Compassion is a good antidote [to empathic distress]," says Klimecki. "It allows us to connect to others' suffering, without being too distressed."[16] Creating a plan for *cultivating compassion* in your own life—whether you bear witness a little or a lot—will go a long way in both preventing and healing from empathic distress. (Social support is also key for reducing empathic distress, so be sure to maintain a community and diverse network of support. See Stage Six—Finding Your Tribe—for more.)

The loving-kindness practice the researchers chose for their subjects is an ancient method for developing compassion. It comes from the Buddhist tradition, but it can be adapted and practiced by anyone, regardless of religious affiliation. Creating a daily loving-kindness practice can be invaluable, especially if you're dealing with *primary* trauma stress—if you participate in direct animal rescue, witness animal abuse, work in an animal medical clinic or emergency hospital, or if you work undercover in some type of animal exploitation facility—but it is also essential if you're dealing with *secondary* trauma stress: the emotional duress you experience when you see or hear about the firsthand trauma experiences of another. You may experience *secondary* trauma if you film or edit videos of animal abuse; if you work on legislation or litigation where you're exposed to visual and auditory accounts of animal neglect and abuse; or if you read,

> Empathic distress is the problem. Compassion is the remedy.

watch, or listen to anything related to animal suffering. In other words, a mindfulness practice will benefit anyone and everyone who wants to deepen their compassion and strengthen their ability to deal with stress, especially stress that can come from being awake in a world that is sleeping. The basic idea is to extend feelings of warmth and compassion in three or four phrases that are repeated throughout a single sitting period. There are no rules, and you can sit for fifteen minutes or fifty, but the more you practice, the more you will benefit. I've included a traditional recitation I've been using for years on page 81, but you can create or find one of your own.

## TOO MUCH OF A GOOD THING?

While empathic distress is a bigger risk for "ethical vegans" who voraciously consume information related to animal suffering, there are also pitfalls at this stage for those who voraciously consume information related to the nutritional benefits of plant consumption and become so fixated on eating healthfully that it becomes an obsession. Reading labels, being mindful of ingredients, and choosing whole foods over processed products are not pathological behaviors in and of themselves; having been conditioned to believe that animal products were essential for optimal health, many of us are eager to make up for lost time. But when you become *preoccupied* with the purity of the food you eat, when *fear* dictates the foods you choose and those you avoid, when you *obsess* over the latest research about superfoods, when you *demonize* whole categories of foods, and when you think that a whole foods plant-based diet is a cure-all for every ailment and disease, the desire for optimal wellness can turn into disordered eating patterns.

In 1997, a medical doctor coined the term *orthorexia nervosa* to describe the obsession with healthy eating he had seen in several of his patients. Built from the Greek *ortho* meaning "straight, correct" and *orexis* meaning "appetite, diet," it translates to "a fixation on righteous or correct eating." *Orthorexia nervosa* is not an official medical or psychological diagnosis, and I'm reluctant to use the term lest it sound like I'm pathologizing healthy eating. After all, healthy eating isn't exactly most people's problem; unhealthy eating is. The most preventable killers in industrialized countries are those that have been coined the *diseases of affluence*—atherosclerosis (hardening of the arteries, which leads to heart disease and stroke), cancer, and diabetes—and all are linked to the consumption of meat, dairy, and eggs. Recent research from the *Journal of the American Medical Association* concluded that diets high in meat and other animal-based protein were associated with a higher risk of premature death, and diets high in plant-based proteins, such as nuts, legumes, and beans, were associated with a lower risk of premature death. Eating more healthfully is a solution—not a problem.

That said, I do think some people can turn the desire for optimal wellness into an obsession. In fact, because orthorexia has less to do with self-esteem and poor body image than with fear of illness and poor health, some experts classify it as a form of OCD (obsessive-compulsive disorder) and say it's seen more prevalently in type-A personalities—people who tend to be more controlling, competitive, and self-critical. There is a line between being health-conscious and being health-obsessed, and it seems to rest somewhere between wanting to eat what's healthy and being *anxious* about eating only what's perceived as "pure." People who view food through this lens of perfectionism take the desire to eat well to the extreme, carefully controlling their diet, feeling virtuous for eating only "clean" foods, feeling polluted if they eat something "unclean," and experiencing anxiety over not being able to eat perfectly all of the time.

> There is a line between being health-conscious and being health-obsessed, and it seems to rest somewhere between wanting to eat what's healthy and being *anxious* about eating only what's "pure."

To be clear, just because you diet, avoid allergens, honor your food preferences, eat mindfully, or characterize yourself as "plant-based" or "vegan" doesn't mean you're unhealthily fixated on gastronomical purity.

Nor is that the case if you avoid certain food groups because of allergies or medical conditions such as celiac disease. However, allergies and ailments aside, when it gets to the point that you denounce any recipe and fearfully avoid any dish that contains even trace amounts of oil, sugar, salt, soy, carbohydrates, wheat, gluten, or alcohol, the road to health can look more like drudgery than joy. When the "good foods" list keeps getting shorter and the "bad foods" list keeps growing, when the guidelines become rules, when the rules become unbreakable—it may be time to stop and take stock.

Aside from the psychological distress this type of rigid eating can cause, it can also be socially and personally disruptive, leading to any of the following situations:

- avoiding eating out with friends because you're afraid the restaurant won't have menu options healthy enough for you
- avoiding eating anything made by anyone else because you don't know exactly what the ingredients are
- identifying so strongly with your diet that you avoid associating with others who don't eat the way you do
- avoiding any "processed" food for fear it will make you unhealthy
- avoiding common allergens, such as soy or wheat, not because you're allergic to them, but because you consider them unwholesome
- overattributing every physical ailment to something you ate (or didn't eat) or to something you eat once in a while
- flitting from one plant-based diet trend to the next, such as low-fat, high-carb, high-protein, calorie-restriction, fruit-only, water fasts, etc.
- feeling virtuous or morally superior to others because of how purely you eat
- feeling guilt or self-loathing for not being perfect, especially when you compare yourself to others you think *are* perfect, such as "influencers" you follow on social media

Rigid eating is seen in many health-conscious communities; it is *not* specific to those who abstain from animal products. And some people mislabel anyone who eliminates specific foods—including vegans— as being rigid eaters. But it's important to remember that rigid eating isn't simply about restricting certain foods; it's about how an individual adheres to a particular way of eating and the way they *use* restrictions to foster disordered thinking and behavior around food.

I've included rigid eating in this first stage—voracious consumption of information—because it is indeed the voracious consumption of nutrition-related information and videos that can contribute to obsessing over being healthy. Consuming books, articles, and social media feeds and photos about healthy eating and living can be motivating and inspiring, but it can also lead to feelings of inadequacy and guilt. Continuously scrolling through picture after picture of perfectly toned, barely dressed, mango-eating, smoothie-drinking men and women flexing their muscles or stretching their limbs in downward facing dog is enough to make the most self-confident feel self-critical. Healthful living has become a competitive sport in its own right, as we track the calories we eat, the steps we walk, the miles we run, and the calories we burn as a matter of course and, for some, a matter of control.

> Consuming books, articles, and social media feeds and photos about healthy eating and living can be motivating and inspiring, but it can also lead to feelings of inadequacy and guilt.

Just as overconsuming information related to animal exploitation can lead to anxiety and burnout, so too can obsessing about being healthy. While neither is beneficial in terms of long-term happiness and well-being, there is evidence to suggest that individuals in the latter group may be at a greater risk of recidivism than those in the former. A study published in the journal

*Appetite* on the "differences between health and ethical vegetarians" found that people who are vegetarian for ethical reasons are more likely to remain vegetarian than people who go vegetarian for health reasons.[17] Is it because ethics are a stronger motivator than health? Is it because "ethical vegetarians" (and vegans) are more aware of animal suffering? Is it because "health vegans" don't see veganism as part of their identity (see Stage Six)? We don't know for sure, but having a rigid view of what constitutes healthy eating may be one reason.

Two possible explanations for self-described "health vegans" returning to eating meat, dairy, or eggs are eating a calorically restrictive diet and having unreasonable expectations about the healing power of plant foods. Another study in *Appetite* found that health-motivated vegans were less likely to take either vitamin B12 or vitamin D supplements, possibly because they believe that whole plant foods are a superior source of essential nutrients and that supplements are artificial and thus "impure." If that's true, it may place health-motivated vegans at higher risk for nutrient deficiencies, and it may also be the reason they return to eating meat, dairy, or eggs (and feel better once they do). It's not that eating a whole foods plant-based diet isn't optimal in terms of health and wellness, and of course no reputable doctor would recommend substituting dietary supplements for healthy plant foods, but nutrient deficiencies can be caused by any number of factors (hormones, stress, malabsorption, digestive issues) and may not always be remedied by whole foods alone. (In other words, supplements may help.) The bottom line is if you expect veganism to be a panacea for all your health issues, you're more likely to attribute any new hard-to-diagnose ailment or possible nutrient-related deficiency to the fact that you've stopped eating meat, dairy, and eggs. Add to that obsessive googling, getting nutrition advice from the unaccredited University of YouTube, and following ex-vegans on social media, and chances are you'll stop being vegan.

Taking charge of your own health isn't inherently bad, but when speculation supplants science and diet trends take precedence over common sense, being your own diagnostician can be a slippery slope. If you become convinced that it's more "natural" to get your omega-3 fatty acids from eggs or fish rather than from a supplement (even though, these days, egg-laying hens and farm-raised fish get their fatty acids from supplements added to their feed), you're likely to start eating eggs and fish again. You may even feel better once you do so. It's possible, however, that you would have also felt better if you took omega-3 supplements made from algae (the origin of omega-3 fatty acids) while continuing to eat a whole foods plant-based diet. The same applies to eating a calorically restrictive diet (which many ex-vegans admit to adhering to): if you're perpetually lethargic, hungry, and unable to concentrate, it may be because you aren't getting enough fuel (that is, calories) to sustain your energy and mental acuity. If you add meat, dairy, and eggs back into your diet—and thus more calories—you will most likely feel more energetic, satiated, and clear-headed. It's possible, however, that you would have felt just as energetic, satiated, and clear-headed if you just ate more calorie-dense plant foods.

> When speculation supplants science and diet trends take precedence over common sense, being your own diagnostician can be a slippery slope.

Eating enough calories, having reasonable expectations about the healing power of food, and redefining what healthy eating looks like are just a few of the ways to counteract the negative effects of overconsuming health-related information and thus feeling the temptation to return to eating meat, dairy, and eggs. Here are some more:

◆ If you're struggling with disordered eating or depression, low self-esteem, or body image issues around food and eating, consider seeking help from a professional, such as a cognitive behavioral therapist.

- Find reliable sources for health information, but keep in mind that even experts don't have all the answers—including nutritionists, dietitians, naturopaths, acupuncturists, and medical doctors. New studies, data, and research are published all the time, and some will contradict former conclusions. But just because nutrition advice is fluid doesn't mean there aren't key foundational concepts that remain constant.

- Don't believe the hype. If something sounds too good to be true, it probably is. Use common sense and have a measured outlook.

- Lower your expectations. Plant-based eating/veganism isn't a cure-all for every ailment. That means you will get sick, have colds, and be susceptible to nutrient deficiencies—just like non-vegans. There are numerous health advantages to treating and preventing those illnesses and deficiencies with plants, but you don't stop being human when you become vegan. Sometimes additional help (such as supplements) may be needed. It doesn't mean you're failing as a vegan; it means you're accepting that you're human.

- Be discerning. Just as people can have unreasonable expectations of veganism's ability to prevent all illnesses, they can also over-attribute health issues to plant-based eating. There are so many factors when it comes to wellness: stress, pollutants in the air and water, social relationships, alcohol intake, smoking, sleep, exercise, and many more. Diet is only one component, so if you're having health issues, take a holistic approach and examine other areas in your life that might be contributing.

- Think broadly. When people ask me if a "vegan diet" is healthy, I have to ask them to clarify what a "vegan diet" is. There is a huge spectrum of *how* to eat vegan, and there are thousands of edible plant foods. Not all of them will agree with you. Not eating meat, dairy, and eggs leaves open hundreds of possibilities of what and how to eat, so if you're eating one way as a vegan and feel you need to make changes, then make changes within the context of remaining vegan. You don't have to throw out the baby with the bathwater if something isn't working for you. Maybe you need more plant protein or iron or calories. Maybe you need more sleep, exercise, sunlight, or micronutrients. All of that can be achieved without eating animal products. You may be sensitive or allergic to a particular food. You may feel better when you eat at particular times of the day. You're not a failure if you don't like beans, or they make you feel bloated or break out. By the same token, if you discover you're allergic to strawberries, that doesn't mean you need to drink cow's milk. You may just need some time, some adjustments, and possibly some medical or nutritional advice and support.

- Incorporate some kind of mindfulness practice into your life, such as the Loving-Kindness Meditation recommended on page 81.*

- Practice mindful eating, which is all about having a positive relationship with food—eating with full attention and awareness and savoring with all your senses every bite you eat.

- Consider taking a moment before you eat to express gratitude. Just taking a moment to give "thanks" is a form of mindfulness. Do it silently or say it out loud, but speak from the heart. Something I say each night before my husband and I eat is: "We're grateful for the food in front of us, the love between us, the roof above us, and the animals among us." Feel free to use this, or create your own.

Bearing witness takes courage, but it also requires self-honesty: knowing how much you're able to bear before becoming distressed. It means looking without staring, participating without dwelling, caring without

---

\* For more on eating mindfully as a vegan, check out Lani Muelrath's book, *The Mindful Vegan*.

becoming a martyr. Bearing witness takes strength, but it also requires self-regulation, including choosing to stop participating in what causes the distress in the first place, as needed. This may mean taking a break from the kind of intense activism that requires exposure to violence against animals, whether in person or through visual media. It might mean taking a break from reading health blogs while working toward having a more relaxed relationship with food and eating. Self-compassion means creating boundaries, taking a break, keeping expectations in check, and developing stress-reduction practices such as these ten, which have been scientifically and historically proven to be effective:

> Bearing witness takes courage, but it also means looking without staring, participating without dwelling, caring without becoming a martyr.

1. meditation
2. deep breathing exercises
3. sharing your emotions with trusted loved ones
4. muscle massages
5. laughter
6. guided imagery (of soothing scenes or animals)
7. soothing music
8. physical exercise (running, walking, yoga, etc.)
9. repetitive mantras or prayers
10. making a gratitude list

While any and all of these strategies can be implemented in *response* to the tension and trauma of bearing witness, they will be more effective if they're part of your regular routine. Incorporating stress management into your daily regimen will make you more resilient and less likely to burn out or give up in the first place.

# Loving-Kindness Meditation

The original name of this practice is *metta bhavana*, which comes from Pali, a language native to the Indian subcontinent and widely used in Buddhist scriptures. *Metta* means "love" (in the nonromantic sense), benevolence, or kindness: hence *loving-kindness*, for short. *Bhavana* means cultivation or development. It's often referred to simply as metta meditation or loving-kindness meditation.

The most common form of this practice unfolds in five stages. Because it's essential that you have compassion for yourself in order to have it for others, it begins with ourselves, shifts to focus on specific people, then extends outward to include all living beings. Gradually, both the visualization and the repetition of four simple phrases combine to create a feeling of loving-kindness. The more you practice, the more loving-kindness you cultivate.

Take at least three to five minutes for each category.

## Yourself

Sit in a comfortable, relaxed position. Close your eyes, breathe naturally, focus your attention on your heart (and perhaps place one or both hands on your heart), and recite silently to yourself:

> *May you be happy.*
> *May you be safe.*
> *May you be free of suffering and sorrow.*
> *May you be at peace.*

You can modify the words to those that most open you up to giving and receiving compassion. Repeat several times, letting the words penetrate your heart and mind and experiencing the sensation of loving-kindness throughout your body.

## A loved one

Next, picture someone who is close to you, someone you feel comfortable being around, someone you feel a great amount of affection for—a loved one, an animal, a dear friend. Notice how it feels to think of them. Perhaps you feel a sensation of warmth, joy, and tenderness. Imagine these feelings filling every cell of your body, and while you're imagining your loved one sitting in front of you, extend those sensations to them—from your heart to theirs. Silently repeat:

> *May you be happy.*
> *May you be safe.*
> *May you be free of suffering and sorrow.*
> *May you be at peace.*

Continue repeating these phrases to yourself silently, all the while imagining those sensations of warmth, joy, and tenderness projecting from your heart to theirs.

## An acquaintance

Next, visualize someone you don't know very well—someone you neither strongly like nor dislike, but who you see in your daily life, such as a neighbor or coworker or classmate you're not familiar with, a store clerk, mail carrier, or a stranger you pass on the street. See them in your mind's eye. Although you don't know them very well, imagine how this person may suffer in his or her own life. Perhaps they have conflicts with loved ones or struggle with an addiction or illness, or have been the victim of trauma, violence, or loss. Imagine a situation in which this person may have suffered. Pay attention to the sensation in your heart. Perhaps you feel warmth, openness, or tenderness. Allow these feelings to fill every cell of your body, and while imagining this person sitting in front of you, extend these sensations to them as you silently repeat:

> *May you be happy.*
> *May you be safe.*
> *May you be free of suffering and sorrow.*
> *May you be at peace.*

## A foe

Next, visualize someone you have difficulty with in your life or in the world. This may be a parent you disagree with, an ex-partner or friend, a coworker you don't get along with, an animal abuser you read about, a slaughterhouse worker, or a hunter. Although you may have negative feelings toward this person, think of how this person may have suffered in their own life.

Contemplate the fact that this person has had conflicts with loved ones or has suffered illness, abuse, trauma, or loss. Think of a situation in which this person may have suffered. Now, bring your attention to your own heart. Imagine this person sitting in front of you as compassion wells up in your heart. Extend it to theirs. This may be difficult to do. Simply be aware of the sensations you feel. Perhaps it's warmth, openness, or tenderness. Perhaps you feel sadness, anger, or an aching sensation. Just be aware of these sensations, and imagine compassion in your heart filling up and extending to their heart. Imagine that compassion imbued with warmth and joy, peace and tenderness; imagine that it is easing their suffering.

Silently recite and repeat several times:

> *May you be happy.*
> *May you be safe.*
> *May you be free of suffering and sorrow.*
> *May you be at peace.*

## All beings

Now direct your loving-kindness toward everyone—yourself, the loved one, the acquaintance, the foe, the animals, everyone. Recite and repeat several times:

> *May all beings everywhere be happy.*
> *May all beings everywhere be safe.*
> *May all beings everywhere be free of suffering*
>   *and sorrow.*
> *May all beings everywhere be at peace.*

You may linger on each section for as long or as short as you like, but even a few minutes combined can make a difference. Fifteen to twenty minutes is a typical length of time for a loving-kindness meditation, but one study showed that even just a single seven-minute loving-kindness meditation "made people feel more connected to and positive about both loved ones and total strangers, and more accepting of themselves."[18] Imagine what a regular practice could do! And you don't have to be sitting down with your eyes closed to practice it. Sometimes, when I'm just outside walking around in a public place, I silently repeat the meditation's phrases to each person I see: *May you be happy. May you be safe. May you be free of suffering and sorrow. May you be at peace.* I repeat them silently to passersby, to store clerks, to little critters I see, or to folks who look like they could really use a dose of compassion. It may not change them, but it certainly changes me.

*Stage Two*

# Guilt, Regret, and Remorse

*Finding Peace and Choosing Self-Forgiveness*

Remorse begets reform.

—William Cowper

I f our principal questions in Stage One are *How can this be happening?* and *How can this be real?* then the questions we ask in Stage Two are *How could I not have known? How could I have participated? How could I have let this happen?* and *How could I have been part of this?* When I first started formulating these stages, I never had any doubt that this would be one of them: a deep feeling of regret over past behavior we were unaware at the time was causing harm—harm to ourselves, harm to animals, harm to our children, harm to the environment. Originally, I characterized this feeling as *guilt*, but I soon realized there's more to it than that.

Earlier, I discussed the fact that while we were consuming animal-based meat, dairy, and eggs,* we chose ignorance over awareness—however many times our conscience reared its head, urging us to wake up. In favor of social conformity and conditioning, however, we kept our conscience at bay by justifying our behavior as being both necessary and beneficial, by accepting industry marketing campaigns as truth, by minimizing facts, by trusting biased corporations to be reliable sources for nutrition information, and by undermining our own values and goals. Rather than yield to our conscience, we gave into our blindness by denying any feelings of guilt. In other words, guilt was underneath our discomfort all along. If we didn't feel there was something problematic with eating meat, dairy, and eggs in the first place, we wouldn't have worked so hard to justify our behavior, and we wouldn't have tried so hard to avoid looking at the processes and consequences of what we were paying for. *Don't tell me. I don't want to know* is not what we say when confronted with how carrots are harvested from the ground or how plums are plucked from trees. *Don't tell my children what they're really eating. It would be too upsetting for them* is not what we say when asked about how

> *Don't tell me. I don't want to know* is not what we say when confronted with how carrots are harvested from the ground or how plums are plucked from trees.

---

* The word *meat* originally referred to any food—not simply the flesh of animals for consumption—and we still use that meaning today in sweetmeat, coconut meat, and nut meat. That is why I distinguish between plant-based and animal-based meats—to make that point and reclaim the word.

apples become applesauce. In all aspects of our life, guilt serves as a red flag that something isn't right, tapping us on the shoulder to let us know we may have strayed from our principles or goals.

And that's a good thing. That is to say, whereas our *conscience* is our moral compass, our *guilt* is the discomfort we feel when we violate our moral code. Guilt can drive us to do the right thing or stop us from doing something we know is wrong, unethical, harmful, or unhealthy. Guilt can compel us to change our behavior or make us feel enough discomfort to stop us from repeating an offending behavior. *Guilt* is one of the reasons many people become vegan in the first place. Being kind to animals and not intentionally causing them harm is part of the moral code most of us live by. Eating animals creates guilt, because—even though we avoid facing it directly—we're aware that animals suffered for our benefit. I've received countless emails over the years attesting to this. Here are just a few:

"I started getting a gnawing feeling (which was my guilt) for not living the values I hold so highly (namely compassion)."

"I remember listening to your Food for Thought podcast a few years into being vegetarian and feeling uncomfortable, guilt-ridden, and defensive when you would talk about veganism. I even (regrettably) skipped episodes where I thought you would be talking about dairy. Finally, something clicked and I couldn't ignore my guilt any longer."

"I thought I was doing the right thing for my health (and my kids' health) eating meat and especially dairy. After all, that's what we're taught! But I also know that I avoided looking at the truth because I felt too guilty. I knew if I delved deeper, I wouldn't be able to deny anymore that being vegetarian (and eventually vegan) was the best thing for me and my children."

"I was an omnivore before starting my vegan lifestyle. I always felt immense guilt when eating flesh or animal secretions. It always felt wrong but I was scared that I would not have the willpower to move over to a vegan lifestyle and so I made a whole lot of excuses to make myself feel better."

Many people also talk about the sense of relief they feel upon transitioning—a sense of peace that comes from reflecting their deepest values, or their desire for optimal wellness, in their daily behavior. I can vouch for this personally, and it is also something I've heard from countless vegans.

"I can now look into the eyes of my two rescue cats and my shelter pup and not feel guilt or shame. I'm now living according to my values, and I've found peace."

"Once I became vegan, I couldn't believe how happy and light I felt. I no longer felt the constant guilt that stemmed from contributing to the abuse and death inherent in the meat and dairy industries. Since becoming vegan, I've felt much more connected to the Earth and all the creatures we share it with."

"My husband and I joyfully became vegans two months ago. We have never felt better. This has been a wonderful transformation for us— most of all because we no longer harbor guilt over what our two-year-old son currently eats (and will eat in the future). This journey started out as primarily for health purposes but quickly reflected our deeper moral systems."

"Freeing myself from the constant guilt of contributing to the slaughter of so many innocent lives and the related environmental consequences has given me a peace that I never thought possible."

"I feel that some kind of weight has been lifted off my chest. Like there was some guilt accumulating in my body for years and now I am releasing it."

"I'm newly vegan now, and this lifestyle that for so long seemed too restrictive and extreme is something I'm so excited about. There's no more guilt, no more excuses. It's freedom. The relief you feel is amazing—the calm that sits inside you, the absolute joy that sometimes overwhelms you. I still giggle at the idea of calling myself a 'joyful vegan' . . . but it is just so appropriate."

Peace of mind is indeed a byproduct of becoming vegan. It is an unexpected gift. The guilt we felt while we were eating animals is all but gone. However, that is not necessarily the end of the story for everyone. Some vegans then reflect on all the animals and animal products they once ate and feel bad for not having done something about it sooner. *How could I not have known? How could I have been part of it?* At first glance, this looks like guilt, but it's really something much deeper: *remorse*.

*Guilt* is what we felt when we were eating animals (which manifested in our willful blindness, excuses, and justifications).

*Remorse* is what we feel when we *stop* eating animals and reflect on how blind we were and how much damage we caused—to the animals, to the environment, to our own health, and to the health of our families.

*Regret* is also a word people use, especially when describing how they wish they had stopped eating animals sooner, and I think it's worth unpacking the difference between *regret* and *remorse* as well—and why the distinction matters.

*Regret* is feeling sad or sorry about something that you did or did not do.[1]

*Remorse* is a gnawing distress arising from a sense of guilt for past wrongs.[2]

Actually, the image of being *gnawed at* is a fitting one because the word *remorse* comes from the Latin word *remordere*, which means "to bite again." When you're feeling remorseful, you feel its bite *again* and *again*. You keep picking at the same wound over and over—never giving it a chance to heal.

*Regret* is less intense than remorse, and it tends to encompass emotions ranging from disappointment to sorrow because of something you or someone else did or didn't do. *Remorse* is typically felt only about something *you* did or didn't do, and it is characterized by self-reproof and self-reproach. You feel *regret* over something relatively minor, but you feel *remorse* when you're aware that you violated your moral code—even if it was unintentional. Remorse is directed inward, causing a nagging feeling of distress over a mistake or a lapse in judgment—usually one that resulted in harm. Getting on the other side of remorse entails admitting your error and taking responsibility for the consequences, which is another way it distinguishes itself from regret or guilt; when you're remorseful, you have a desire to *repent*, to make *amends*, to *repair* the wrong you have done.

Like guilt, remorse can also be healthy in that it demonstrates that you're capable of feeling sorry for having caused pain or suffering; it means you're capable of recognizing the difference between right and wrong or appropriate and inappropriate behavior. Remorse is one of the barometers society uses for determining antisocial behavior or psychopathy. To be remorseful is to be capable of self-reflection and introspection and, in this way, remorse is a healthy reaction. In fact, in the Western justice system, *perceived* remorse—being able to determine that someone feels bad about what they did—is one way judges and juries assess offenders during trials, sentencing, and parole hearings and in restorative justice.

However, while the ability to feel remorse is a sign of a psychologically healthy person (or of one who has the potential to reform), when remorse turns into self-condemnation or prolonged self-flagellation, it can be harmful. If we let remorse consume us, it can lead to depression and self-loathing, and that's not good for anyone—ourselves or the animals.

Now, I have to reiterate that not everyone who becomes vegan or plant-based will go through this stage. The stages I'm identifying are not prescriptive, so not everyone goes through each and every one; you may not feel any remorse at all, and that's perfectly fine. You don't *have* to; it's not a requirement, and it's optimum if you don't! But even if you don't experience this stage yourself, remember that identifying these stages is as much about helping you help others through the process as it is about helping you through it. Even if *you* don't experience remorse for your pre-vegan actions, you may meet someone who does, and with awareness of this stage, you'll be able to tell them that it's a normal part of the process.

> If we let remorse consume us, it can lead to depression and self-loathing, and that's not good for anyone—ourselves or the animals.

## GUILT WHILE VEGAN

Having made a distinction between guilt and remorse—the former being what we feel *while* we're eating animals (and their eggs and milk), the latter being what we feel as we reflect upon *once having* eaten animals—I do think there is one way we experience *guilt* even once we've stopped eating animal flesh and fluids, and that is when we beat ourselves up for not being perfect, such as in these situations:

- ♦ when we eat an animal product by accident
- ♦ when we become obsessed with eating as healthfully and "purely" as possible (see the discussion of rigid eating in Stage One)

- when we realize that we still own sweaters made of cashmere, blankets made of wool, comforters and pillows made from feathers, coats made from down, neckties made from silk, shoes made of animal skins, and car seats or furniture made of leather
- when we unintentionally hurt animals, perhaps by hitting them with our car or bicycle

As we enter a way of living whereby we consciously strive to do our best to avoid hurting animals, of course we feel terrible when we fall short—or when someone else judges us for not being perfect. The worst is when that judgmentalism comes from other vegans—usually in the form of the self-appointed vegan police—who tell you you're not a "real vegan" for these or other reasons:

- You eat peanut butter made on equipment that was touched by dairy products.
- You feed your (carnivorous) cats meat from aquatic or land animals.
- You eat (vegan food) in nonvegan restaurants or with nonvegan friends.
- You stopped eating animal flesh and fluids for health rather than ethical reasons.
- You buy your produce from traditional farms that use animal products to fertilize the crops.
- You eat white sugar (which is sometimes filtered through bone char), palm oil, nonorganic fruits and veggies, and genetically modified foods.

Sadly, with the increase in the number of people becoming "plant-based" for health reasons (not "vegan" for ethical reasons), there has also been an increase in the forming of factions within a community that should be celebrating similarities rather than dwelling on differences. I discuss this more in Stage Six—Finding Your Tribe—but it's worth noting here, because the propensity for judgmentalism and guilt-mongering is seen on all sides:

♦ Those who are vegan for the animals condemn those in the "plant-based" community for not going further and shunning animal products in their clothing as well as in their diet.

♦ Those who call themselves "plant-based" criticize and sometimes mock vegans for not being "healthy," for eating "junk food," and for being overweight or unfit.

♦ Those who became vegan for the animals knock "dietary vegans" for not being activists.

♦ Vegans censure people who call themselves "99 percent vegan" because they're not 100 percent vegan.

Of course, most of this shaming takes place online, where it's easy to attack in the comfort of anonymity, but it takes place in person as well, particularly at vegan events and conferences. Some people argue that a little judgmentalism is necessary, because some things are abusive, illegal, or immoral. After all, if we don't judge when things are ethically wrong, how would we function as a moral society? How would we create laws and rules of conduct? Well, of course we need to determine when something is wrong and then act accordingly; having a moral compass doesn't mean we don't make evaluations and create consequences for offending behavior. But, there's a difference between *making a judgment* and *being judgmental.* There is a difference between *being discerning* and *being judgmental.* The bottom line is there is no such thing as a licensed vegan. No vegan is perfect, and if you perceive being vegan as being an end in itself—as if it's a goal to attain, a club to join, a milestone to reach, or a badge to wear—guilt will plague you. Being vegan is not an end in itself; it's a means to an end.

> Being vegan is not a goal to attain, a club to join, a milestone to reach, or a badge to wear. There is no such thing as a licensed vegan.

Ironically, those feelings of frustration at imperfection may very well result in someone giving up entirely and returning to eating animal products. Many ex-vegans say they went back to eating meat, dairy, and/or eggs rather than feel guilty about not being a perfect vegan. (Many also say they felt guilty because they were berated for being imperfect—by other vegans!) This is terribly unfortunate, because returning to eating animal products rather than accepting that the world isn't black and white is completely self-defeatist. For the sake of the animals we want to help and the health we want to attain, we absolutely must shift our perception and recognize that veganism is inherently imperfect. That is to say, *imperfection is built into being vegan* because *imperfection is built into being human.*

> Imperfection is built into being vegan, because imperfection is built into being human.

There's no denying it can be upsetting if you eat an animal product by mistake or if you accidentally hurt or kill an animal, but that is just part of being human—of trying to live consciously in an imperfect world. *Let it come, let it be, let it go.* Learn from it, move on, recalibrate, and remember why you became vegan in the first place. If you have cashmere sweaters, silk ties, wool blankets, or shoes, car seats, or furniture made with leather, as you're able to replace them, you will. As you become less comfortable with animal products in your home and on your person, you will slowly eliminate them from your life. It's all part of the process. Just as *becoming* vegan is a process, so is *being* vegan. If you're unable to afford replacing them or if you're not the only one making this decision (perhaps your car is under a lease or a family member loves the leather sofa), the question we might want to ask ourselves is: *How does keeping this couch [for instance] contribute to animal cruelty?* Or flipped around: *How does getting rid of this couch help animals?* The answer to those questions may help you decide what to do next or at least enable you to forgive yourself and alleviate your guilt.

Living an examined life means learning to tolerate the gray areas we inevitably encounter. Accidentally consuming an animal product, wearing old leather shoes until they wear out, or keeping our grandmother's pearl earrings doesn't make us *less* vegan. It just makes us *more* human. Imperfect humans in an imperfect world using this thing called veganism to reduce harm and illness is a pretty fantastic way to reflect our values of compassion and wellness. It should enhance our life—not diminish it. So, whether we're feeling guilt or remorse, these are the questions we need to ask: How do we move through and get to the other side? How do we not let it consume us? How do we make reparations for the harm we feel we caused? How do we advocate for animals while remaining emotionally healthy ourselves? How do we strive to be healthy while accepting we are also fallible? I think the answer to all of these questions is *forgiveness*.

## FORGIVENESS

Many people have a tendency to cling to guilt, remorse, or shame because they think—unconsciously—that by letting go, they are tacitly condoning whatever it is they feel guilty, remorseful, or shameful about. They accept remorse as penance for the suffering they've caused, as if perpetual guilt will make up for the mistakes of their past. I see this play out when vegans are reluctant to forgive themselves for having once consumed animal flesh and fluids—the implication being that forgiveness would mean condoning that behavior. Many who become vegan for the animals feel as if, by letting go, they are "letting the animals down." Health-oriented vegans navigate their own guilt—especially if they're dealing with a food-related illness or a disease they learn they could have (possibly) prevented had they become vegan sooner. *The biggest misconception about forgiveness is that it condones the offending behavior and leaves the door open for future infractions.* I think another reason vegans are reluctant to forgive themselves for having contributed to animal suffering is because it would mean they would have to forgive *others* for continuing to do the same. In other words, a certain amount of martyred satisfaction comes with remorse, but *forgiveness* is the way out (that is, *if* you want to get out, and not everybody does).

> Many people have a tendency to cling to guilt, remorse, or shame because they think—unconsciously—that by letting go, they are tacitly condoning whatever it is they feel guilty, remorseful, or shameful about.

Strictly speaking, *to forgive* is "to grant pardon without harboring resentment, to refrain from imposing punishment on an offender." Etymologically speaking, *forgive* is a compound word composed of the Old English prefix *for-*, meaning "completely," and the Old English word *giefan,* meaning "to give."[3] Whether the recipient is the self or another, whether forgiveness is asked for or not, and whether it is deserved or not, forgiveness is all about letting go. It is not about condoning or overlooking bad or harmful behavior; it's about *choosing to be unattached to the guilt or remorse that accompanies it*—whether that guilt is your own or the guilt you believe someone else should feel. Choosing to forgive doesn't mean you come away with positive feelings about the offense, necessarily, but it does mean you let go of the negative feelings associated with it.

But the first step in letting go—of getting on the other side of remorse—is to be *willing* to let go. Moving beyond negative emotions means being *willing* to move beyond them. However unpleasant they may be, negative emotions can become habitual or even addictive. They can become part of our identity, which makes letting go of them more challenging and even scary, so the first thing we need to do is figure out how guilt and remorse serve us, then determine if we're even *willing* to let go of our attachment to them. The following questions may help:

→  How does this guilt/remorse serve me? What am I getting out of it?
→  How does this guilt/remorse help or serve animals?
→  Do I want to continue feeling bad about something I did in my past?
→  Does having negative hindsight motivate me to do better now, or am I just chastising myself because it feels familiar? Because it feels good? Because it demonstrates that I care?

Taking some time to answer these questions may help you understand what it is you're holding on to and give yourself permission to let go of it.

Next, we need to identify what exactly we feel remorseful about. As much as we were indoctrinated to eat animal flesh and fluids, we are indeed conscious beings with free will, so it can be helpful to take stock and identify *when* and *where* in the process of eating animals we received signals (i.e., pangs of guilt) and ignored them. In other words, did we have the opportunity to make another choice and didn't? Why? Was it out of fear of not fitting in? Does that still play into our lives today as vegans? Did we find ourselves making excuses for eating animals? Why? What were we afraid of? These questions may serve as a guide to help get to the source of our remorse:

→  Do I feel remorse because I ate animals and animal products and thus contributed to their suffering?
→  Do I feel remorse over being duped? Over being gullible? Over being too naïve or not strong enough to resist indoctrination?
→  Do I feel remorse because I (or someone I love) developed physical ailments as the result of my consumption of animal products?
→  Do I feel remorse because of the habits I instilled in my children, who now have a taste for animal flesh and fluids?

Once we identify exactly what we're feeling remorseful about, the next step is being open to having a new perception of ourselves and our experience.

So, to recap, the first step is *determining why* we've been attached to remorse, the second step is *being willing* to let go of that remorse, and the third step is *getting clear about* what we feel remorseful about. The fourth step is *beginning the process of forgiving ourselves*. Self-forgiveness is about taking responsibility but also about understanding our actions in the context of a larger perspective. Forgiveness is about realizing we are only human and being clear about what we have control over and what we don't. It's about understanding that our perception of the past is only in our minds, and by changing our minds, we have the power to change the past. In letting go of our attachment to our past and to our guilt, we will feel lighter and better able to live in the present.

The fifth step in letting go of remorse is the act of *making amends*.

## MAKING AMENDS

We can't turn back the clock, but there is much we can do to move forward, and certainly the greatest restitution we can make lies in our decision to become vegan. It feels good to have aligned our daily behavior with our deepest values, and that is reason enough to celebrate. So is the fact that by being vegan, we are accomplishing so much:

- lowering the demand for animal products in the marketplace
- increasing the demand for vegan products
- decreasing the number of animals raised and killed for consumption
- offsetting environmental impacts
- improving our health
- inspiring others around us

No wonder we feel peace of mind.

Being vegan may be your way of making amends, and it's enough—and a lot—if that's all you do. Period. Full stop. However, some people may want to take extra steps to compensate for the past, and there are many gestures you can make to do so—gestures that are symbolic as well as concrete. Whether you call them reparations, restitution, amends, or atonement, these positive actions not only help in the process of letting go, they also disrupt patterns of negative thoughts and perceptions that may be weighing us down. Choose one, some, or all of the following suggestions to help move beyond remorse.

1. **Keep things in perspective.** We all do the best we can with the information we're given. When it comes to our consumption of meat, dairy, and eggs, all our lives, on a daily basis, we're bombarded with messages to eat as much of this stuff as possible, so it's no surprise that we do. To continually punish ourselves for not having known or even for having chosen willful blindness is futile and slightly masochistic. Even in the criminal justice system, one of the basic tenets is that the punishment should be proportionate to the crime. You don't get twenty years in prison for running a red light. Forgiving ourselves means taking responsibility for behavior that we recognize as having caused harm, but it also means not overmagnifying that behavior.

2. **Apologize.** A sincere apology consists of an admission and an expression of regret not for the results of an action but for the action itself. Note the difference between "I'm sorry you were hurt by my actions" and "I'm sorry my actions hurt you."

   *To the animals:* We obviously can't directly apologize to the individual animals we ate and whose milk we drank and eggs we consumed. So making amends might entail making a *symbolic* apology. While this apology may not make a difference to animals, it can make a difference to *us.* You can make amends in writing or silently in your mind.

   *To yourself or loved ones:* Similarly, it's not always possible to apologize directly to a person you feel you may have hurt, and you can't undo the past. If you feel that your past eating habits caused you or your loved ones to experience illness, you can make amends by apologizing either directly to them or silently to yourself. I hear from a lot of parents who didn't know any better but to feed their children animal products and who now feel guilty that their children don't want to eat or don't know how to prepare healthier plant-based foods. This is an opportunity to take responsibility for the past and move forward into the future.

Regardless of who your recipient is, start by finding a quiet spot. Close your eyes, envision the animals, yourself, or other recipient of your amends, and find the words that are authentic for you. When you're finished, take a deep breath, and experience the gratitude and liberation that come with releasing such a burden.

3. **Get involved.** I once heard someone say *do good rather than feel bad.* I think that's a perfect way to characterize how present actions can make up for past behavior.

    ***With animal rescue organizations:*** Fostering, rescuing, or adopting animals is a wonderful way to make amends. It may feel more significant for you if it's farmed animals you help directly, but even providing a home to dogs, cats, or rabbits can do the trick (and make a difference to those individuals, of course). If you can't adopt or foster animals, many shelters, sanctuaries, and animal rescue organizations offer volunteer opportunities where you can socialize with, walk, brush, pet, or care for animals in one way or another.

    ***With plant-based health organizations:*** Similarly, there are plenty of individuals and organizations that promote and teach plant-based eating. Volunteer with one of them, or become an independent advocate by teaching vegan cooking classes or influencing your friends and family on social media.

4. **Make a donation.** If you're unable to care for animals or teach people directly—or even if you are—make a donation to organizations that work on behalf of animals or promote plant-based eating.

    *For the animals:* When donating, you can even designate that it be made *on behalf of* or *in the name of* a particular animal. Give a name to an individual animal you may have hurt or killed while driving, or to the animals you ate before you were vegan, and make the donation on their behalf.

    *For a healthy world:* There are many organizations promoting plant-based eating in schools, hospitals, and the general public.

    Identify the organizations you value, become a member, and turn your remorse into support.

5. **"Adopt" or "sponsor."**

    *For the animals:* Many animal sanctuaries and shelters enable you to symbolically "adopt" a particular animal, even providing you with a photo and story of your adoptee. This is a powerful way to transform an anonymous animal raised to be killed into a living animal who has a name, a face, and a history.

    *For a healthy world:* Work with legislators to sponsor specific legislation to make plant-based meals available in school districts, hospitals, and other public institutions. Support an existing bill or help draft a new one. You might even look for organizations that enable you to "adopt a classroom" or "adopt a school," allowing you to focus your resources on helping a specific group of people learn about healthy plant-based eating.

6. **Spend time.**

    *With animals:* If you have companion animals, give them some extra uninterrupted time, take them for an additional walk, play with them a little more. Be fully present with them. If you don't have your own animals, help someone else's. Walk a neighbor's dog, spend time with a friend's cat, ask friends or neighbors if you can help when they're at work or when they go out of town.

*With yourself and your loved ones:* If eating unhealthy animal products or feeding them to your family members is something that makes you feel remorseful, spend time *undoing* those habits. Take a plant-based cooking class on your own or with your family. Start a vegetable garden, make going to the farmers' market a regular outing the entire family participates in, or spend time in the kitchen learning new plant-based recipes that will become part of your repertoire.

7. **Make mindfulness part of your daily ritual.** Certainly apologizing and making amends either directly or symbolically (see #2) may be enough to help you feel liberated from your remorse, but a regular practice of mindfulness enables you to cultivate a mind-set of self-love and compassion.

    *For the animals:* Include animals in your regular mindfulness practice of prayer, meditation, or yoga. The Loving-Kindness Meditation on page 81 includes a section for sending compassion, love, and peace to all beings.

    *For yourself:* Likewise, include *yourself* as part of your mindfulness practice. The Loving-Kindness Meditation also includes a section for sending compassion, love, and peace to *yourself*.

8. **Address related issues.**

    *For the animals:* Wild animals suffer greatly for our consumption of farmed animals. They're killed or displaced for "competing" with livestock, and their habitats are destroyed in favor of crops grown for cattle, poultry, and pigs. Make amends by putting out water for them, reducing the noise or light pollution around your home, giving them a quiet place to raise their young, or making sure they have a corridor behind your home so they can safely migrate. (In densely populated residential areas, animals have lost the ability to move about safely without having to cross dangerous roads.) You can also donate to wild-life rescue/rehabilitation organizations in your area, which can be especially meaningful for you if you've ever accidentally hurt or killed an animal.

*For yourself:* Wellness is not limited to what we put in our bodies; it also includes how we holistically treat our bodies. Challenge yourself beyond what you ever imagined possible for your body, such as by creating some kind of fitness goal or try-ing a new sport. Exercise muscles (literally and figuratively) that you've never used or that you've let atrophy.

9. **Speak up.** We'll cover specific advocacy tips in a subsequent chapter and communication tips in another, but speaking up for animals or about healthy plant-based living is a wonderful way to make amends.

*For the animals:* Most people aren't even aware of the gen-eralizations they make about animals or the language they use that disparages them. You can be a voice for animals by cor-recting misconceptions, sharing positive stories about them, or using compassionate idioms instead of violent ones ("cut two carrots with one knife" instead of "kill two birds with one stone," for example*).

*For health:* When it comes to the health benefits of eating plant-based, there are many misunderstandings about what it means to live (and thrive) without meat, dairy, and eggs. Your voice can help provide and perpetuate a different perspective. Share your knowledge, experience, and enthusiasm.

10. **Share your feelings.** Whatever you do, share your feelings with others. You will find that simply sharing your sadness and

---

* My podcast *Animalogy* is about the animal-related words and expressions we use and how they affect and reflect how we treat and regard animals.

remorse with others will tap into their emotions or experiences. The more we realize we are all part of the same human condition, the more we seek to cause less harm to one another and to the rest of the world.

*For the animals:* When people ask you why you're vegan, don't hesitate to tell them it's for the animals if that is indeed your story. Let the conversation unfold, and be a voice for the animals you care so much about. (See Stage Seven—Finding Your Voice—for more on effective communication.)

*For health:* Ditto when it comes to your enthusiasm for eating plants instead of animals.

Forgiving ourselves for having contributed to the suffering of animals is not only beneficial for ourselves; it's also beneficial for our relationship with others. If we can't forgive *ourselves* for once having habitually eaten animals, we may find that we're judgmental toward others who still eat animals, and that doesn't do anybody any good. If we can't tolerate our own human imperfections, we risk being intolerant of everyone else's, too. This is why it's so important that we *remember our story*. We need to remember that we, too, once ate animals and that we, too, are fallible and vulnerable humans. If we remember that we did the best we could with what we knew at the time, then we will be better able to understand where someone else is at. If we can move through our own remorse to self-forgiveness, it means we're more likely to be compassionate toward others.

*Stage Three*

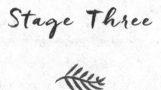

# Coming Out Vegan

## *Explaining the V-Word to Family, Friends, and Yourself*

Human beings are not born once and for all on the day
their mothers give birth to them, but . . . life obliges
them over and over again to give birth to themselves.
—Gabriel García Márquez

magine this:

*You're a new vegan—excited, proud, awake. You skip over to a family member or friend and say, "I love you so much, and I know you love me, which is why I know you'll be thrilled when I tell you I'm now . . . vegan." Your parent (or spouse, sibling, or friend) grabs your hand, does a little jig, and says, "Fantastic! Then I'll be vegan too!" You hug, prepare a kale salad, and make plans to volunteer at an animal sanctuary the next day.*

That's usually how it plays out, right? No? Okay, well then, how about this:

*You casually announce to your friends and family you're vegan; they roll their eyes and say, "Oh no! Please don't be* that *kind of vegan." You backpedal and tell them of course you're not and you insist that you don't expect anyone to accommodate you. You bring your own food wherever you go, downplay your new lifestyle, and dismiss any questions about your diet by saying it's just a personal choice. Everyone feels relieved, and you never really speak of it again.*

No? How about this:

*You worry for months about how to "break the news" to your family. You avoid talking about it at work until you're finally forced to admit it at a networking luncheon where there's nothing for you to eat. You endure jokes about animals being tasty and quips about vegans being unhealthy; you feel attacked, start avoiding certain colleagues, and begin eating alone. When you finally tell your family and friends you're vegan, you brace yourself for the worst, and your fears are realized when your mother asks how you could do this to her and what is she supposed to feed you now. Friends begin sending you articles about how soybeans cause cancer, and acquaintances point out your hypocrisy for still wearing leather shoes. You feel alone, dejected, and resentful; you feel like a pariah among your peers.*

Of course, your exact experience may not be perfectly reflected in any of these scenarios, but perhaps there are elements you can relate to in each. Sometimes the reaction of the nonvegans you come out to is very supportive and affirming, or they sheepishly confess that they eat meat but love animals, opening the door for conversation and camaraderie. But reactions can also range from silence and dismissiveness to defensiveness and hostility to passive-aggressiveness and insensitivity. A vegan doesn't even have to do anything but show up or simply say "I'm vegan" to garner negative responses. And at this stage, we're still raw, vulnerable, and susceptible to attack, so those reactions can really hurt. We've let our guard down, but we haven't yet developed a thick skin.

The point is that *coming out vegan*—telling your nonvegan friends and relatives you're vegan—carries a little more weight than telling them you're changing your hairstyle. Friends and family members don't always respond the way we hope, and new vegans are often surprised by negative reactions they receive. Parents may take it personally and see your veganism as an act of selfishness or as a rejection of them. Friends, neighbors, and acquaintances may grill you with *gotcha* questions. Colleagues and coworkers may challenge you to defend veganism in the context of the history of the world and the evolution of our species, and complete strangers may argue with your reasoning and question your choices. Vegans get the sense pretty quickly that nonvegans wish they would just shut up, go away, and keep their veganism to themselves.

Just a small taste of such reactions may send you running and, indeed, they can shake up even the most stalwart and principled among us. Afraid to rock the boat or call attention to themselves, some people give up entirely and return to eating animal products; some retreat deep into the *vegan closet*, reluctant to emerge lest they be attacked, judged, or ridiculed, and some wish they had never said anything at all for all the trouble and turbulence it causes. Many who encounter hostility upon telling people they're vegan eventually avoid using the V-word altogether, because they're afraid of the reaction they'll get—a coping mechanism that sociologist Erving Goffman called "defensive cowering."[1] In his seminal work on socially stigmatized individuals, Goffman found that one of the ways people protect their identities when they deviate from societal norms is by downplaying the identity that is considered deviant. Although Goffman never explicitly referred to vegans in his work, many parallels can be drawn between the social experiences of the subjects he studied (those considered "deviant" by society's standards) and the typical reactions of vegans in social contexts. Feeling the need to hide such a significant aspect of ourselves can lead to further isolation, depression, social anxiety, and self-consciousness—increasing the likelihood of vegans becoming ex-vegans.

Now, *coming out vegan* doesn't necessarily mean you have to go around wearing a neon sign that says **VEGAN** (unless you want to). If you never tell another soul you're vegan (or vegetarian or plant-based or animal-product-free or however you choose to identify), that doesn't make you any less vegan, but my hope is that you feel proud, stand tall, and speak truth in your vegan shoes without the fear of being judged or the pressure to be perfect. You don't have to announce to the world that you're vegan, but you also shouldn't feel ashamed or apologetic about it or deny or downplay who you are and what you care about.

The process of *coming out vegan* also isn't meant to imply that you were once closeted, oppressed, or stigmatized; it's as much a celebration as it is a revelation of your identity and values. As we discussed in chapter two, new vegans especially tend to feel a sense of peace, a newfound energy, and an overall feeling of relief. Exhilarated by what feels like a rebirth or at least a life-altering awakening, they can hardly contain the joy that comes with living in alignment with their deepest values or experiencing renewed health, and they can't imagine anyone seeing anything negative about their decision. Generally speaking, becoming vegan is a positive experience—mentally, emotionally, and physically—and new vegans are genuinely excited to share their enthusiasm with others, especially the people they're closest to. Although some vegans do closet themselves because they're uncomfortable calling attention to themselves, *coming out vegan* doesn't necessarily mean you've been hiding. It means completely owning who you are—unabashedly and unapologetically. Originally from the world of debutante balls in which young women are presented to society, "coming out" is an apt term to use for our purposes to characterize the celebration of self-actualization.

That is to say, *coming out* is a process that is personal as well as social, and I think many vegans overlook the private work required to move from personal awakening to public revelation. What often gets neglected is the need for self-acceptance and self-compassion. Before we can come out publicly, we need to take time to *define* as well as *claim* our new vegan identity privately. There are vegans who say they don't want to call themselves "vegan" because they don't want to be typecast as *that* kind of vegan—militant, judgmental, angry, or fill-in-the-blank stereo-type. There are people who call themselves "plant-based" in order to distance themselves from the moral implications wrapped up in the word "vegan."* And there are vegans who are ashamed to say they're vegan because they're afraid they're not a good representation of veganism—because they're

> Before we can come out publicly, we need to take time to *define* as well as *claim* our new vegan identity privately.

overweight or underweight, because they have an eating disorder or an acne condition, because they have a chronic illness or they get periodic colds. The amount of pressure society puts on vegans doesn't compare with how hard we are on ourselves. So, let's talk first about how self-acceptance, self-awareness, and self-compassion must be the foundation of our coming-out process. Before we define veganism for others, we need

---

\* If you do eschew animal products for health reasons and call yourself "plant-based" instead of "vegan," in the spirit of promoting a positive perception of your vegan brethren, try to be cautious of not celebrating your identity at the expense of someone else's. In other words, be mindful of not saying, "I'm plant-based for my health. I'm not one of those crazy vegans."

to define it for ourselves. When we do, we are better able to avoid getting caught up in our own misconceptions and other people's projections.

## WHY ARE YOU VEGAN?

I often jest that the most common question vegans hear is *Where do you get your protein?* but in truth, I don't think it is. I think the most common question vegans hear is *Why are you vegan?* And yet very few vegans have an answer to this very basic question—or at least they haven't crafted an answer that is both truthful for them and palatable for others. Taking the time to answer this question for yourself will not only give you clarity about your own values and intentions, it will also enable you to express yourself articulately and truthfully when you tell people you're vegan. I'm vegan because I don't want to contribute to violence against animals—either directly or by paying someone else. Why are *you* vegan?

> The most common question vegans hear is *Why are you vegan?* And yet very few vegans can articulate an answer to this very basic question.

Take time to get your thoughts down on paper or on screen. Practice free-writing or journaling, or use these questions as a guide:

→ What was the catalyst for me to stop eating meat, dairy, and eggs?
→ Do I call myself vegan? Why or why not?
→ Do I call myself plant-based? What does the term mean to me?
→ When did I first hear the word *vegan*?
→ What did it mean to me when I first heard the word? What does it mean to me now?
→ Has my perception of veganism changed over the months or years?

→ What about being vegan has been the most challenging for me?

→ What has been the most rewarding?

The more time you take to work out the answers to these questions, the closer you'll get to a succinct, authentic response to the question *Why are you vegan?* Your reasons may expand and change over time, which is why it's a good idea to revisit your answer to that question every so often. It's not about having the perfect sound bite, but rather about finding clarity and confidence.

In fact, knowing your reasons for being vegan and being able to articulate them is a key factor in remaining vegan—or in sustaining any significant change, according to researchers James Prochaska and Carlo DiClemente. In the 1970s, based on their work studying how people successfully quit smoking, Prochaska and DiClemente devised a model of behavior change called the "transtheoretical model of behavior change" or, more simply, "the stages of change."[2] This model posits that individuals move through six stages when changing their habits and behaviors—precontemplation, contemplation, preparation, action, maintenance, and termination—and just as with the ten stages in this book, movement through these stages of change is not necessarily linear, since people cycle and re-cycle through each one. According to this theory, successful behavior change (that is, sustaining a new habit for two years or more) includes periodically rewarding your progress, reviewing your motivations, and refreshing your commitment to your new behaviors.

If your reasons for being vegan change over time, welcome that, as well.

## VEGANISM IS IMPERFECT

Coming out—celebrating our own vegan identity—means first defining what being vegan means to us. Being vegan isn't about adhering to a set of rules or doctrines; there's no instruction manual to memorize. As we've seen, because many people mistakenly believe that being vegan is about attaining some kind of goal, they often accuse vegans of being hypocrites when their behavior falls short of perfection. Remember: being vegan is a means to an end—not an end in itself—and if we get hung up on trying to be perfect, we'll make ourselves and everyone around us miserable.

> Being vegan isn't about adhering to a set of rules or doctrines; there's no instruction manual to memorize.

Living with integrity in a world that values convenience over ethics and momentary pleasure over wellness can be challenging, because we live in an imperfect world: the rubber in our car tires has the remnants of animals in them; most of those cars are powered by fossil fuels that are destroying wild habitats; we kill insects every time we walk on the ground or drive in a vehicle; many municipal water systems use animal bones as filtering agents; and most plant-based agriculture still condemns vast numbers of wildlife to displacement and death. Clearly, we have to find a line to draw when it comes to striving to live consciously in an imperfect world, or we'll drive ourselves crazy. But just because we can't be perfect doesn't mean we have to be indifferent. We need to continually remind ourselves (and others) that we shouldn't do nothing just because we can't do everything. Doing something can be everything. In other words, define your own veganism in the context of the imperfect world we live in.

## TELL YOUR STORY

It's easy to *become vegan* and forget there was a time you weren't.

As with all of the stages I've identified here, you will return to this one again and again over the years, because every time you tell someone you're vegan, it's another *coming out* moment. By the time you've done some work to articulate what being vegan means to you and how you came to it, you'll be able to answer with confidence and truth when someone asks you why you're vegan. Now, if you're also an activist, you may feel this is the perfect opportunity to enumerate all the peer-reviewed studies, stats, and facts that support the benefits of being vegan (and there are plenty), but from a communications and relationship-building perspective, I'm not so sure that's the best tactic. After all, the question isn't *Can you tell me the benefits of being vegan, making sure to provide footnotes and citations?* I think the most effective thing you can do when someone asks *Why are you vegan?* is to simply tell them why *you* are vegan. They're curious about *your* story, *your* narrative, *your* personal experience. So, tell them. You did the work getting clear about why you're vegan; now take advantage of it!

When someone asks me why I'm vegan, I tell them *my* story, *my* truth, *my* authentic reason for being vegan, which is simply this: *I grew up loving animals and never wanting to hurt them, and when I realized I was paying people to do just that, I stopped.* I tell them, *I don't want to contribute to violence when I have the power and choice to avoid doing so, and when it came to my consumption of animal flesh and fluids and my support of the slaughter industry, I had agency, so I exercised it.* I tell them that *when it occurred to me how absurd and macabre it is that we bring animals into this world only to kill them, I stopped participating in this system.* I tell them that, or some other variation of my truth.

Unlike with stats and facts, nobody can say "That's not true" or "You're wrong" or "That's inaccurate." Nobody can take away *my* truth, *my* story. There's no way to argue with the fact that I don't want to hurt anyone. No one can say to me, "Oh yes you do!" Nobody can take away *your* story, so tell it.

If you get nervous about having the perfect answer, memorizing statistics, or saying the right thing, focusing instead on telling your own story can banish those fears. When you speak from the heart, there is no right or wrong answer, and personal narratives connect with people in a way statistics don't. What's more, information about the benefits of not eating animals will naturally emerge as part of your story, but when offered in the context of a narrative rather than a lecture, people are more likely to hear it—especially if you frame the information in terms of what *you're doing* rather than what *they're not*.

Note the difference between these two responses:

"When I found out that baby male calves are taken from their mothers upon birth and killed because males are useless in the dairy industry, I was appalled. I just couldn't be part of that anymore, so I stopped."

"Did you know that the dairy products you eat cause the murder of hundreds of thousands of baby calves—800,000 to be exact? Ripped from their mother, they're murdered so humans can steal her milk, which is harmful for us anyway and contains pus and blood."*

We can still convey information; it's just that by keeping it in our own story and not attacking someone who hasn't yet experienced the awakening we have, we do so much more effectively. We'll talk more about this when we get to the chapter on advocacy, but there are countless benefits of *telling your story*, including the fact that someone may see their own in yours. Don't be so attached to having all the answers and being the perfect spokesperson for veganism. Just focus on being a perfect spokesperson for *you*.

## YOU ARE WHAT VEGAN LOOKS LIKE

A few years ago, a woman named Tess wrote me an email that nearly broke my heart:

> *I am an overweight vegan and feel embarrassed that I'm not a good representative for the cause. I'm trying my best to get my weight down, but it's*

---

\* This is not to say that facts don't matter or shouldn't be part of what we convey; we should all have a commitment to the truth. The trick is to have an interpretation: a "story" ready to translate the statistics or numbers into a more powerful meaning. This doesn't mean you should drop all numbers and references to research, but rather that you should use them sparingly and always link them to meaning. For instance, instead of "Go vegan for the animals, the planet, and your health!" try "Research suggests that a cold mentality toward animal life, necessitated by slaughterhouse killings, in turn cheapens regard for human life, which leads to more violence in our world," or "Billions of animals are brought into this world only to be killed—that's not who we are."

*a struggle. When people introduce me or when I tell people I'm vegan, I'm immediately embarrassed.*

Fat-shaming is all too common in our culture today, and vegans are as guilty of it as nonvegans. I've received many letters over the years similar to the one Tess sent me, and my response is this: *Being vegan is not a formula for perfection or immunity against being human.* We still have vulnerabilities, frailties, and idiosyncrasies, and we still succumb to all the challenges and foibles that come with being human. You will *not* turn into a perfect, flawless superhuman when you become vegan. However, you *will* become a more fully realized version of yourself—if you allow it. *You* being who *you* are is the best representation of veganism. *You* being the most authentic, compassionate, kind, healthy, principled, imperfect, well-intentioned person you can be is the best ambassador for veganism, because *that's* what vegan looks like.

> You will *not* turn into a perfect, flawless superhuman when you become vegan. But you can become a more fully realized version of yourself.

Vegans are as diverse as the general population. We come from all backgrounds. We come in all shapes and sizes. We are as varied in style and form as we are in appearance and personality. We can't try to fit ourselves into a mold because there is no mold. Some people assume all vegans are thin. Some assume they're all fat. Some people assume all vegans are sickly. Some are envious of how healthy vegans look. Some people think vegans are all angry. Some think they're pacifist peaceniks. Some people accuse vegans of being extreme. Some criticize them for not going far enough. We can't try to represent for the person standing in front of us what they think "vegan" should look like. What about the person standing behind her and the one behind her? Everyone has a different notion of what "vegan" looks like, and if you try to fit one of them, you'll quickly learn that you're not fitting others. You will *never* please everyone, so you might as well please yourself. Accept yourself as the vegan you are.

Fear of not living up to expectations of what a vegan should look like doesn't come only from stereotypes shaped by nonvegans. Vegans also find that they're judged by other vegans once they come out. There's an expectation—even among vegans—that we can't be fat, we can't get sick, we can't be weak, and we can't ever say we're hungry. When a vegan doesn't fit another vegan's notion of what vegans should look, act, talk, or vote like, she's accused of not being a "real vegan," a figurative excommunication of sorts. I think this stems from the fear among some vegans that individual vegans who don't fit their mold of what vegans should be like will make all vegans look bad, so by *metaphorically* revoking individuals' membership to the vegan club ("They're not *really* vegan anyway"), they will keep the pool pure and the image untainted.

Unfortunately, what really happens is that it keeps the pool rigid in ideology and small in size. When a group is dominated by criticism and condemnation rather than support and solidarity, people don't tend to stick around—or join in the first place. And so a rhetorical banishment becomes an actual exodus, adding to the already high percentage of former vegetarians and vegans. Am I saying it's the fault of judgmental vegans that people become ex-vegans? Let's just say vegans deal with enough pressure living in a nonvegan world, so it certainly doesn't help when members of their own community, in which there is a shared value and expectation of compassion, add even more strain. *Nobody* likes to feel judged.

So, as we contemplate our own process of *coming out*, we must recognize that acceptance—of ourselves and of others—is tantamount to staying vegan and manifesting compassion.

## SEEING THE OTHER SIDE

When I first became vegetarian, my parents reacted the way many parents do; they took it personally and asked, "What's wrong with the way we raised you? You never had a problem eating what we fed you. Why do you have a problem with it now?" Undeterred (but shocked they could even *think* my being vegetarian had anything to do with them), I carried on. By the time I became vegan, I was eight years older and three thousand miles away. Consequently, my being vegan didn't really affect our day-to-day interactions, which may be why, this time, they were generally supportive. Moved by my concerns and persuaded by the same facts about the ill effects of animal agriculture, my husband was incredibly sympathetic and became vegan about six months after I did. So I was most surprised, when I became vegan, by the defensive reaction of some old friends, who had known me for years, supported my being vegetarian, and were keenly aware of my aversion to violence against animals. Their reactions ranged from confusion and defensiveness to silence, and some of these friendships deteriorated. I thought I had handled my announcements with tact and grace, but as I reflect back on that time, I wish I had known then what I know now: that when we become vegan, it can *rock people's worlds.* Just knowing that much can make all the difference in how we interact with and come out to our loved ones, especially in the beginning.

When I *came out vegan*, not only was I oblivious to that fact, I was also embarrassingly naïve. It simply didn't occur to me that anyone would be anything other than thrilled by my being vegan. I figured they'd at least be supportive—and certainly not surprised, given my sensitivity, compassion, and history of animal advocacy. To me, becoming vegan felt like a natural progression. To them, it felt like a slap in the face. And that's what shocked me. If I had at least been aware that my becoming vegan would affect my friends and family so deeply, I would have been prepared. Instead, I was surprised and wounded by their reactions, but I quickly understood why *coming out*—when done without preparation or proper forethought—can put a bit of a strain on relationships.

I'm not suggesting that we anticipate negative reactions. Far from it—I think we should expect the best of people and give them the benefit of the doubt in all circumstances. But I am suggesting that we be sensitive, compassionate, and sympathetic to how changes we make inevitably affect those around us. After all, as we are right now, we are a known quantity—and likely have been for decades. We are familiar. We are predictable. Our friends and family members know who we are, what we believe, and how they relate to us. They've invested heavily in the person they know *at this moment*; they may have even helped shape who we are—especially in the case of parents or siblings. If we change, what would it mean for them? What would it mean for the relationship? Will they still know you? Will they still understand you? Will they have to change, too? What if they don't change? What if they don't become vegan? Will you still be compatible? Will you judge them? Will you still love them? These are some very real concerns with some very high stakes.

I liken this process to a dance. Imagine two people who have danced the waltz together for several years—maybe even decades. They predict each other's steps, they read each other's body movements, they speak each other's rhythmic language. Other than a flourish here and there, there are no real surprises, and both dancers are completely in sync with one another. Now imagine that one of the partners decides to start dancing the steps of the tango. No warning. No sign this change was coming. No comprehension as to why this might upset her long-time dance partner, who is perfectly content with the waltz they'd been dancing all these years. Feeling misunderstood and disappointed that her old partner doesn't want to learn the tango, the tango dancer starts dancing with other tango dancers. The waltzer feels confused, abandoned, and even resentful of the tango. He doesn't stop caring about his old dance partner; he just wants her back. Alas, he doesn't speak the language of tango, and they eventually drift apart.

Humans are creatures of habit and fans of familiarity, and our friends and family members resist change as much as we do, especially when they feel it's foisted upon them when they were perfectly happy with the way things were—when they want to dance the waltz and you're already dancing the tango. Add to that the feeling that not only is their way no longer relevant for you, you may actually see their actions as harmful, cruel, or unhealthy. Why *wouldn't* they be defensive? I think one of the things we forget when we come out to our family and friends is that we've already processed our awakening. We've moved through Stage One, where we've read books or watched documentaries, so we have some pretty strong convictions by the time we actually *come out* to them. They haven't consumed the information we have, but we act as if they have.

Because our loved ones have not been privy to the same information we've been immersing ourselves in, they're looking at the world through a completely different lens and hearing your announcement from a completely different perspective—possibly even an opposite one. I said earlier that I thought I came out to friends and family with grace and tact, but thinking back on those early conversations now, I'm not so sure. I think I made a lot of presumptions about their beliefs and mind-set.

Like a child who lacks the ability to recognize where she ends and another person begins, I probably assumed that friends and family members would share my aversion to meat, dairy, and eggs as soon as I told them how awful eating them is for animals or how dangerous it is for their own health. It didn't occur to me that they were perfectly happy eating meat, dairy, and eggs and didn't at all share my disgust for animal flesh and fluids. In other words, I talked to them as if we were all on the same page. It didn't occur to me that we were at different points on our journey or that our paths might not be crossing anytime soon.

If we expect our loved ones to respond to us with patience, understanding, and compassion, we have to show them the same. Give them time. Give them space. Answer their questions. *Ask* them questions. If their concerns are about your health, talk about it together. If they act defensive because they feel that you're questioning the way they raised you or judging the way they eat, talk about that. But however they react, let them react. Give them time to process your veganism just as you've had time to process it. And be patient—with them and with yourself.

## KNOW YOUR INTENTION

It can be such an emotional time when you first become vegan. You see animal products everywhere you look, and you just can't get certain images out of your head. Though there was once a time when you could look at a burger and just see dinner, now all you see is suffering and sickness. The pain of awareness is so acute, and your sensitivity is unexpectedly heightened. As a result, you may take offense at everything that's said to you, or you may unintentionally offend someone else. The first thing to remember when communicating about this sensitive subject is exactly that: *it's a sensitive subject to communicate about.* It can make people defensive, emotional, irrational, fearful, angry, and dismissive. It can also make them feel guilty.

One of the most awkward *coming out* moments for me occurred just a couple of weeks after I became vegan—when I was a *raw* vegan, and I don't mean I was eating only uncooked fruits and vegetables! I mean that I was emotionally fragile. We had made plans with some old New Jersey friends who had recently moved to California, and I had decided to tell them at the beginning of our date that I was now vegan—as was our home. (David hadn't become vegan yet, but he was supportive in keeping a vegan home.) Our friends arrived at our apartment with milkshakes in their hands—milkshakes made with cow's milk. I vividly remember them sitting on our loveseat, uncomfortably clutching their cups while I stood above them and told them how upsetting it was to have animal products in the house knowing what I had learned about the cruelty in the dairy industry. Not knowing anything about my transformation prior to this, they felt terrible and asked if they should leave since they had milkshakes. I told them of course not—that they didn't know prior to coming over that I was going to make this announcement—but I just wanted to tell them for future reference.

Making my friends feel bad was not my intention, but I'm pretty sure that's what I accomplished. If I could do it over again, I would do things differently. I would have told tell them under neutral circumstances (when they weren't in the middle of consuming animal products) and on neutral terrain (when we weren't in our home). I would have been more sensitive to the tension this subject creates between vegans and nonvegans, and I would have gotten clear about my intentions prior to our meeting. Being clear about our intentions means knowing what we're setting out to do before we do it. Of course, how people react to what we say, what we do, or how we live is not ours to control, but there is a difference between someone feeling bad because of something we said and our setting out to make someone feel bad because of something they did (or are doing). These days when I tell someone I'm vegan, I make sure in my mind that I'm clear about my intention, and that my intention is to *tell my story and to speak my truth.* If my truth upsets someone, that's not for me to worry about, but I never intentionally set out to upset someone. There is a difference, and if we're honest with ourselves, we know when we're doing one versus the other. Good relationships with others are grounded in self-awareness.

## BE SENSITIVE TO TIME AND PLACE

*When* we come out also matters. Imagine again being that new vegan— excited, proud, and awake. As you're about to sit down to dinner with your mother, father, husband, wife, brother, sister, or friend, you announce that you don't eat meat, dairy, and eggs anymore and that you're now vegan. Your parent (or spouse, sibling, or friend) gives you a confused look and replies with one of the following responses:

"Why are you disrupting dinner like this? How can you be so selfish?"

"You always loved my chicken à la king."

"What am I going to make for you now?"

"What's wrong with the way I raised you?"

"How would your poor grandmother feel knowing you'll never eat her special macaroni and cheese with bacon bits again?"

"Don't you know it's not healthy?"

"How are you going to get protein?"

"You always take things too far."

"That sounds awfully extreme."

"Well, I'm sure you are vegan—whatever that means—and I'm also sure you'll eat the meal I went to the trouble to prepare."

"I'm not going to change just because you've changed. You can make your own meals from now on."

And so on. Surprised by their reaction, you react in one of a number of ways:

"You never support me. I should have known this would be no different."

"Animals are being tortured, and you don't even care."

"You don't understand. Why can't you just try to understand?"

"Why can't you accept me?"

"How can you be so selfish?"

"Being vegan is better than contributing to animal cruelty. At least I'm doing something. At least I care."

"You're the one who's responsible for all the misery animals endure. I'm not paying people to torture animals."

And so on. Tensions mount, emotions rise, old unresolved issues emerge, dinner is ruined, and relationships are strained.

If someone is in the middle of eating animals or their secretions, they're going to be less inclined to hear about how harmful these things are—whether from an ethical, environmental, or health perspective. It doesn't mean they won't react defensively even if they're *not* eating animal products, but chances are they'll be less guarded if they're not in the middle of eating meat, dairy, or eggs. Food doesn't have to be avoided entirely when you're telling someone you're vegan; enjoying a delicious vegan meal together is a great way to casually bring it up and disarm them at the same time. Happy bellies and dancing taste buds make for great conversation companions, and as your friend or family member realizes that the fabulous food they just ate was 100 percent plant-based, they also gain a new perspective about what vegan food is.

THEM: That was delicious! What was it?

YOU: Thank you. I'm so glad you liked it. It's a new recipe I never tried before, and everything was vegan! Isn't that amazing?

THEM: You're kidding!? I had no idea vegan food could be that tasty. Are you vegan now?

YOU: Yeah, it's been a couple months, and I feel really good—in every sense: mentally, physically, emotionally.

THEM: Wow. Is it hard? It must be hard.

YOU: The hardest part was getting the courage to watch a documentary about animal agriculture. I'm still learning and changing some new habits, but it just feels right.

And the dialogue begins. It's light, it's casual, it's almost matter-of-fact. Food can disarm people, which helps in such a situation, but because of our attachment to and association with certain foods, such situations can also be loaded with emotion.

## PARENTS MAY TAKE IT THE HARDEST

Frankly, no matter what your age, parents need time to adjust to your lifestyle. They've seen you go through phases and fads, and they may think this is just another one, so they may not take it seriously. Know your story. The clearer you are about why you're vegan, what it means to you, and what it entails, the more you're able to help them support you. If you're wishy-washy, unclear, or inconsistent, you're just feeding their perception that this is a temporary fad that will pass.

Like all of us, our parents are creatures of habit. They have most likely been cooking the same meals for you day after day, year after year; they've gone through your picky phases, they've cut the crusts off your bread, and they've made special meals to accommodate your preferences. Even when we no longer live at home with them, our parents continue to make the same holiday meals for us or our favorite dishes when we visit. They've connected with us through food for years, and now you're telling them that everything is different; it's no wonder they react emotionally. For all these reasons, *let them have their reaction, and remember that it has nothing to do with you.* On one hand, they probably genuinely don't know what to feed you, thinking "vegan food" is something different than what they're familiar with. If they've been making your favorite meals for decades, they're not exactly going to be enthusiastic about changing the repertoire.

On a much deeper level, though, I believe that one of the reasons parents take our veganism personally is because they've used food from the day we came into this world as a way to physically nourish and emotionally nurture us. When we reject the food they've chosen to feed us, it may feel like we're rejecting them and their affections. They may defensively ask, "What's wrong with how we raised you? You always loved the food I made for you! How can you do this to me?"—as if our being vegan is a judgment of their parenting skills. Tell them you understand how different this must be for them and thank them for teaching you to be an open, compassionate, thoughtful person—all of the qualities that led you to make these new choices. Tell them how much you appreciate all the years they've spent feeding you and buying your favorite foods. Tell them this is not just another temporary fad; tell them why this means so much to you. Show them that you're serious. Be consistent. Tell them you need their support and that you're willing to help make it easier. Then help make it easier by showing them

> When we reject the food our parents have chosen to feed us, it may feel like we're rejecting *them*.

what you've learned. Try to remember that there was a time when you didn't know about all the ways to make delicious, familiar meals with vegetables, fruits, grains, beans, lentils, mushrooms, herbs, and spices. Explore together.

Beyond food as sustenance, your parents might be genuinely concerned that you're not going to get all the nutrients you need. Remember, they've been reared in the same pro-meat/dairy/egg culture you have. So, don't just brush off their concerns, tell them they're brainwashed, and say they know nothing about nutrition. They probably don't, but *neither did you before you did*. Validate their concerns and help alleviate their fears. How you do this depends on your relationship with and the personality of your parents. Some parents feel like anything you tell them about *what they don't know* or *what they didn't teach you* is an assault on their intelligence or parenting skills: "I'm the parent here. *I'm* the one who raised *you*." So, be sensitive to those concerns and try to have a dialogue rather than teach a lesson. Some parents are open from the get-go and happy to read or watch what you recommend, so give them some resources and invite them to talk to you if they're interested. Either way, step back, let them process it all, and let them set the pace. Remember, you're not giving them this information to "convert" them (unless they're genuinely asking for that). You're just giving them information to speak to their concerns.

# IF IT WASN'T THIS, IT WOULD BE SOMETHING ELSE

Some parents and family members get upset when you *come out vegan* because they're afraid you'll turn your back on the traditions they instilled in you and the culture in which they raised you. I hear from a lot of people who say, "I really want to be vegan, but I come from a traditional [Italian, Mexican, Spanish, Thai, Vietnamese, Irish, African American, fill-in-the-blank] family. My grandmother would kill me if I didn't eat her [fill-in-the-blank] dish." I address the notion of embracing your various identities in Stage Six, but for the purposes of *coming out,* I want to speak to what it means to be independent, autonomous, self-governing human beings. That's what growing up is all about—becoming separate from our parents, thinking critically, and questioning what we are taught. Rarely do we incorporate everything our parents teach us into our own lives. We reject some habits and traditions and embrace others. We take on some of their beliefs and leave others behind. In the end, we are amalgamations of our parents—not clones. In other words, if it isn't veganism that puts you at odds with how you were raised, it will be something else. Perhaps you differ from your parents or grandparents in terms of politics or religion; perhaps they disapprove of the music you listen to, the major you chose, or the career path you've taken. Differentiating yourself from your family doesn't mean you're rejecting them; it means you're forming your own identity. That's what autonomy is.

In his eight stages of psychosocial development, Erik Erikson describes the stages through which a healthy developing human should pass from infancy to late adulthood. He identifies the second stage as *autonomy,* which takes place between two and four years old. I think it's safe to assume you've already gone through this stage, but it's worth emphasizing what autonomy means in the context of the process of *coming out vegan.* According to Erikson, the existential question at this stage is *Is it okay to be me?* This is when children seek to separate themselves from their parents and experiment with their own individuality; when they realize they're separate people from their parents with their own desires and abilities; when they realize they have the capacity and ability to make their own independent choices—all of which become a source of emotional strength.

Though we may not be able to recall having gone through the autonomy stage as toddlers, it's something we can revisit now as adults. We can consciously exercise autonomy and assert our individuality now as we continue to find those places where we end and our loved ones begin. We can tell our loved ones that we value them for giving us a foundation on which to stand and that *from* that foundation we will create our own. We can say to our parents, "You raised me to appreciate my family, and I do. You instilled in me the importance of appreciating our traditions and the history of our family, and I honor that. You taught me the value of caring about others, doing the right thing, and thinking critically, and because of that, here I am. My being vegan isn't a *rejection* of what you taught me. It's an *extension* of what you taught me." They still may not accept your being vegan right away, but conveying your appreciation for the values they taught you even as you assert your autonomy is a kind and compassionate approach to what can sometimes be an emotionally fraught experience.

## THINGS DO CHANGE

One of the friends I called after I became vegan had been a mentor to me back in New Jersey—a mother-figure who shared my love of animals (she volunteered for a greyhound rescue) and accommodated my pescatarianism and then my vegetarianism over the many years I knew her. Because I was so raw in those early days after reading *Slaughterhouse* and because I considered my friend to be a fellow animal-lover and compassionista, I couldn't wait to share my news with her, and I'm sure I didn't hold back in telling her how upset it was for me to learn about the atrocities in the dairy and egg industries. I don't remember exactly what I said, but

I know I shared my sadness and outrage over how terrible it is for cows raised for dairy and hens raised for eggs, and I declared that as a result I *became vegan*. She responded with a very noticeable silence, then a staccato "hmm," then an apathetic "wow," and then . . . she changed the subject. It hit me in the gut. I didn't expect her to do cartwheels, but I suppose I expected support and understanding and basic *interest* in what I shared. When we spoke again, I talked about the activism I was doing for animals, and she continued to show little interest. Perhaps it was the geographical distance that now separated us, perhaps it was because she projected that I had changed, perhaps it was her own guilt—I don't know, but after that, our friendship started petering out and eventually withered away. It made me sad then and still does today, but indeed even the best of friendships don't always stay the same.

The truth is, your coming out may very well end a relationship. Over time you may just stop relating to one another, you may become disenchanted with each other, or the friendship may just fade in intensity. You may experience a lull and return to one another at a later time. Relationships change. While this is a part of life, in the context of *coming out vegan*, there's a little more to say.

In section one, I talked about all the reasons people want us to stay asleep: they don't know how your being vegan is going to change you or your friendship or your perception of them, and that scares them. The unknown scares them. They want things to remain as they were. Perhaps food was a significant part of your relationship (it is for so many); perhaps you ate out together, cooked together, shared recipes, tried new restaurants. When you tell them you're vegan, they may be afraid this will change. They may also be afraid that you're going to judge them, try to convert them, or try to change them. And it could be this fear that makes them retreat. Here's my suggestion for alleviating their concerns about your trying to convert them: *don't*.

I made mistakes when I first *came out vegan*, and you will too, because we're not perfect and because we're passionate and earnest about not causing harm. Once you wake up to the violence being perpetrated against animals day in and day out, you can't help reacting with what might seem like zealotry to others. Even when your motivation is wellness, when you become awakened to the healing power of foods, it's hard not to point out the disease-causing foods all around us. I'm not in any way suggesting that we quell our enthusiasm, but I *am* suggesting that we express our enthusiasm with thoughtfulness and with no intention other than to share something important with those we love. In other words, be joyful, be excited, be sincere, be authentic, speak for animals, speak about whatever it

> Be joyful, be excited, be sincere, be authentic, speak for animals, speak about whatever it is that motivates you, but do so without using it as a platform to convert someone else or deliberately make them feel bad.

is that motivates you, but do so without using it as a platform to convert someone else or deliberately make them feel bad.

We'll talk about this in subsequent chapters on communication (Stage Seven) and advocacy (Stage Nine)—about the importance of planting seeds and remaining unattached to the outcome—but for now, let me say honestly that even if you do this perfectly, I can't promise that you will be able to alleviate all of the fears of your family and friends. Things may not stay the same. *You* may not stay the same—you've already changed, in becoming vegan—and that's not necessarily a bad thing. It's just different, and of course, *different* can also be scary. Honesty and frankness are the best approach for addressing these concerns—and being as kind, compassionate, and open as possible. That doesn't mean you should walk on eggshells, accept abuse, or *stop being vegan* to please others or to alleviate their fears, but just holding the perspective that they may be feeling vulnerable or insecure will perhaps enable you to feel less rejected and more sympathetic.

An email I received from a woman named Melissa beautifully expresses this paradigm.

*I have to tell you that for many years I have struggled with "excuse-itarianism." Since I was a teen (and I am now thirty-eight years old!), I have struggled with staying vegan. My excuses have been couched in real challenges, but that is just what they were. Challenges. Not roadblocks. And, honestly, I have been using those real challenges to justify succumbing to underlying fears about what it might mean for me to really commit to being vegan. Last night, on my way home from work, I was listening to your podcast when it hit me. All of my excuses have masked an underlying insecurity in me. I can blame my inability to commit to being vegan on gluten intolerance, digestive issues, or whatever, but the reality is that I haven't wanted to speak up! I haven't wanted to "speak my truth," as you so eloquently put it. I haven't wanted to make waves by asking for what I need. I have been afraid of how others might perceive me—"needy, high-maintenance, difficult, crazy"—if I say, "I'm vegan," I have to face the possibility that others might judge me in these ways. I have been afraid of being hurt. I have been afraid of being judged. I have been afraid of being an outcast, of being "the other." What I realized last night is that I have been putting my fear above the love and compassion I have for other beings—human and nonhuman. This is not OK with me! Is it going to kill me if someone thinks I am a pain in the butt? No! But it will kill somebody if I don't speak up and say no to the consumption of animals. . . . In order for me to really be vegan, permanently, I have to be willing to get vulnerable. I have to risk someone not liking me, or feeling "put out" by me. I have to find and use my vegan voice. But this is a small price to pay for living a life of authentic compassion.*

*As I contemplate this new responsibility, I am also aware of the potential for freedom and empowerment in the work of finding and using my voice. It has been my experience that while getting vulnerable and taking responsibility can be scary and hard, it ultimately leads to a more expansive state. It leads to better relationships, not worse. It leads to more depth, more authenticity, and more love and compassion. The world needs this. The animals need this. I need this. I am ready for the next chapter in my life. I am no longer an excuse-itarian. I am a vegan.*

Keep living your life, speaking your truth, and demonstrating the kind of compassion you would want in return, and trust that nothing remains the same and that's okay. Change is in the nature of things. Birds molt their winter feathers, stars explode, trees drop their leaves, winds change their course, people change their minds—and their behavior. The way your existing community members react to you when you first take on this new identity is not how they will always respond. As they recognize that your being vegan is just one of the many facets of who you are—if not the

> Keep living your life, speaking your truth, and demonstrating the kind of compassion you would want in return.

manifestation of the *best* of who you are—they will adapt. When they discover that you still accept and love them for who *they* are, they will become less threatened and more relaxed. Things get better. We grow, we mature, we expand—as long as we're open to it.

## Keeping a Vegan Home

According to the aforementioned Faunalytics survey on recidivism, about one-third of ex-vegetarians and ex-vegans said they were living with a nonvegetarian/nonvegan significant other when they started eating meat again. Of course, just because we live with people who eat meat, dairy, and eggs doesn't mean we can't stay vegan, but if we don't feel supported in our own homes, if we aren't comfortable asking for what we need, if we don't feel a sense of belonging, it can make a huge difference in our ability to remain vegan—not to mention *joyful*. Here are some suggestions for navigating the social and emotional aspects of extending your personal values into your home when you're not the only one in it.

### I want to keep a vegan home, but my partner/loved one does not. What do I do?

As with any issue in a relationship that causes tension, communication is key. Express yourself clearly, compassionately, openly, and honestly about why you don't want animal products in the house. Speak from the heart, then listen with compassion and openness. Be flexible and willing to compromise and find a solution you can both live with.

Here are some options for meeting each other halfway:

- No animal *flesh* is allowed in the house, but dairy-based cheese and eggs are permitted.
- Meat, dairy, and eggs are kept in a separate refrigerator.
- Meat, dairy, and eggs are permitted in the house (perhaps still in a separate refrigerator), but meat isn't *cooked* inside the house. It's cooked either outside, such as on a grill, or it doesn't require cooking at all (such as lunch meats).

None of these are perfect solutions—each requires someone to bend—but relationships are all about compromise. The idea is to find a solution that works for everyone.

### How do we tell friends, family, and neighbors we don't want animal products brought into our home without sounding rude?

This is why *coming out vegan* to people in your life is so important—and doing it with grace and sensitivity. Telling people you keep a vegan home doesn't necessarily have to be a big announcement; it will most likely come up in casual conversations and when you extend invitations to others. Over time, people will just know. However, to avoid any misunderstandings once they arrive, direct communication is always best.

Whenever we host dinners, parties, or potlucks (and we host *a lot*), we include on the invitation that if our guests want to bring something, we ask that it be free of meat, dairy, fish, or eggs. (Not everyone knows what "vegan" means, so be specific.) I usually add a postscript telling them I'm happy to offer suggestions or vegan recipes if they need any. People appreciate knowing what's expected of them. These days, people tend to be mindful of allergies and dietary preferences, so making such a request is really not that unusual.

Have there been situations when people have brought animal products over—either by mistake, or because they didn't realize our home is vegan? Yes, absolutely. Did we freak out? No. As clear as we try to be, there will always be situations in which animal products make their way into our home, and we handle each situation as best we can—with grace, tact, and kindness.

Are there people who resent that we ask them to bring only plant foods into our home? Are there people who think we're rude? Are there neighbors who don't come to our house because of it? I have no idea. I've experienced only positive reactions from people. Many are even excited to bring vegan dishes they've never made before—and many bring dishes made from recipes in my cookbooks! Of course, I'm not aware of what people say about us when we're not around, but neither do I have any control over their opinions. Some people keep a kosher home; some keep a peanut-free home; some keep a shoe-free home (we do!). Drawing boundaries based on religion, health, or cleanliness is no more or less valid than drawing boundaries based on ethics.

Our home is our refuge, our sanctuary, our haven. There's a lot we can't control in this nonvegan world, but if we can't draw that line at our own front door, then where can we draw it?

## Stage Four

# Evangelism and Fundamentalism

## *Knowing the Difference Between Enthusiasm and Zealotry*

Do your work, then step back. The only path to serenity.
—Lao Tzu (trans. Stephen Mitchell), *Tao Te Ching*

There's a universal joke that goes: "How do you know if someone is vegan? Don't worry. They'll tell you." On the one hand, it's true. Vegans do talk about being vegan a lot of the time—especially new vegans, whose altered view of the world informs everything they see and say. On the other hand, vegans often talk about being vegan because they're asked to. "Why are you vegan?" is, as we've already acknowledged, one of the most common questions vegans are asked, and it's often elicited merely by the *presence* of a vegan—a phenomenon I call *being the vegan in the room.* Although some vegans lament that they're expected to explain why they're vegan while nonvegans are never asked to account for the fact that they eat meat, dairy, and eggs, the truth is, many people are genuinely curious about what inspires someone to *become vegan.* And so they ask. And we answer—often with strong emotions and great passion.

How can we not? Having had a significant shift in the way we live our lives and in the way we see the world, it's only natural to want to share that experience. Sharing enthusiasm brings us closer to the people in our lives, it validates us, and it makes us feel good. In fact, findings from a recent study conducted at Brigham Young University suggest that just the *act* of sharing happiness boosts well-being.[1] When we recount a positive experience to someone and receive in return encouragement and support, we feel more happiness, love, and appreciation. When the response to our positive news is apathy, negativity, or criticism, we feel deflated and dejected, which can lead to anger (see Stage Five). This is certainly the case for many vegans, who innocently share their excitement about their transformation only to be met with defensiveness, rejection, and accusations of being didactic, pushy, or evangelistic. In many cases, the vegan is just sharing their enthusiasm (often in response to inquiries). In some cases, however, they're actively proselytizing. The stereotype of the preachy vegan is well established, and it deserves some attention.

## VEGANGELISM

When I tell people that I've identified this stage in our vegan journey as evangelism (or, better yet, *vegan*gelism), I'm met with a little laughter and a lot of head-nodding, because everyone knows exactly what I mean. Especially when we're newly vegan, we're excited, we're passionate, and we want everyone to experience the same enthusiasm (or at least know about ours). This isn't to say that vegans are never preachy and didactic (I've reserved the second half of this chapter to discuss just that) or that raising awareness about violence against animals isn't necessary or shouldn't be part of our advocacy (more about that in Stage Nine), but what I'm referring to here is the genuine excitement we feel having become awake—the passionate expression of "Oh my word! I had no idea, and now that I know and my life is changed for the better, I want to shout it from the rooftops!" It's the desire to share the good news, which is exactly what *evangelism* is and exactly what an *evangelist* does.

The word *evangelism* comes from the Greek word *euangelion*, meaning "to bring good news." (In early Greek Christian texts, *evangelist* was the name given to each of the four writers—or "messengers"—of the narrative gospels in the New Testament: Matthew, Mark, Luke, and John.) Etymologically speaking, an evangelist is literally "a messenger of good news," but because it's often equated with the religious dogma of Evangelicals and conflated with proselytizing and fanaticism, negative connotations weigh it down. The assumption is that if you're an evangelist for something, your primary goal is to convert others to your cause, whatever that may be. Thus, anything that smacks of passionate zeal has become suspect in many people's eyes, and ardent enthusiasm inevitably gets equated with fanatical zealotry, especially if people feel they are being sold something or are being told what to do. So, when vegans appear overly enthusiastic in proclaiming the numerous benefits of veganism, they're often disparaged as being evangelical—in the negative sense of the word. The solution, however, isn't to stifle our passion, hide our

> We can be enthusiastic without being overzealous, informative without being didactic, knowledgeable without being preachy, and persuasive without proselytizing.

excitement, or silence our voices. We can be enthusiastic without being overzealous, informative without being didactic, knowledgeable without being preachy, and persuasive without proselytizing. The question is *how*? I think the answer lies in awareness, intention, and memory; it's the difference between drawing people in and pushing people away.

1. **Have awareness.** As I emphasized in the chapter on *coming out vegan*, we need to be aware of the fact that people are beholden to their beliefs; if you even appear to be telling them that they're wrong or that they need to change, they will not only be turned off by those insinuations, they may be even more protective about their beliefs/behavior. Just knowing that people are sensitive to being preached at or being "converted" is a good start, and it will help you remember that their reaction usually has nothing to do with you personally. The topic of veganism can bring up feelings of guilt, discomfort, or sadness in others; just by being *the vegan in the room*, you're reminding them of the dissonance that so many of us experience and try to squelch (as discussed in section one). That's not to say you should distance yourself or withhold the truth of who you are from others, but it does mean at least *understanding* that your presence may evoke strong emotions and irrational responses.

2. **Share your news, then stop.** If we embrace the positive aspects of evangelizing—spreading the word, sharing the news, raising awareness, and genuinely, authentically, and unabashedly expressing enthusiasm—we can have a very positive experience when we talk about being vegan. If you approach every situation with the intention to share your news without being attached to the outcome, you will have many constructive interactions, indeed. (I discuss this at length in Stage Seven, on communication.) Some readers may interpret this to mean that we should water down our message and temper our passion, but that's not what I'm saying at

all. We should absolutely be clear about our message (including if it's about animal suffering) and present it with passion and enthusiasm (if that is indeed how we feel), but the trick is to be unattached to how the message is received—whether it's received negatively or positively, whether someone changes as a result or not. That's not your business. That doesn't mean someone won't still mistake your passion for proselytizing, but that's also not your business. If you are genuinely expressing excitement about something and being clear in your mind about your intention, then how someone responds is not your burden to carry.

3. **Avoid oversharing.** Try to read the person you're talking to and identify signals that indicate they might be annoyed, defensive, restless, or bored. Let there be silence. Let there be pauses. Even if they've asked *you* for information, people can take in only so much, and no doubt you have a lot to share. Less can definitely be more, and if you've conveyed your message with compassion, kindness, enthusiasm, and humor, the person you're speaking to will be more apt to absorb and recall it, especially if you're not overwhelming them with figures and statistics. In fact, research suggests that people are less inclined to remember the specifics of what you *say* and more inclined to remember how they *feel* being in your presence.[2] If they associate you (and veganism) with *hope* that they can make a difference rather than *shame* that they're doing something wrong, that will add even more weight to whatever specific facts you share with them.

4. **Vegangelize. Don't proselytize.** It may seem like I'm splitting hairs, but in the decades I've been doing my work guiding people to becoming vegan, I've never once said "go vegan"—not in my podcast, not in my books, not in my social media posts. And yet, I hear from countless people every month who tell me they've become vegan because of my work. Of course everything I do is to promote the message of compassion and this thing called

*veganism* as the way to manifest unconditional compassion and optimal wellness, but since my intention is to raise awareness about violence against animals and give people the tools and resources they need to live compassionately and healthfully, I've never had to tell people what to do. I might encourage them to take the 30-Day Vegan Challenge so I can provide support and inspiration, but that's still different from telling someone to "wake up" and *become vegan*. Asking someone to "go vegan" is a tall order, and as a vegan advocate, it means your success or failure is dependent on that person changing both their worldview and their behavior. We all know how hard it is to change our *thinking* about something, and we know how it is equally difficult to change our *behavior*. There's a difference between expressing how much I love being vegan and saying "and you should be vegan, too." It's the difference between being an evangelist (one who shares a message) and a proselytizer (one who tries to convert). It's the difference between being enthusiastic about your beliefs and dictating that others should live by them.

5.  **Remember your story**. Ironically, the awakening we experience can also give us amnesia. Having awakened, it's easy to forget that we were once unaware. In sharing our story with others, we need to include the parts of the tale that preceded our becoming vegan or "plant-based." In recalling and recounting our own cognitive dissonance, our own resistance to change, and even our own affinity for the taste of meat, dairy, or eggs, we're more inclined to make connections with other people. Because nonvegans may already have their defenses up, bracing themselves for a sermon, they probably don't expect to have anything in common with you. Sharing the fact that you, too, once enjoyed eating animals will give them something to identify with and aspire to—*If you can do it, so can I*—rather than feel that their situation is unique and that change isn't possible.

# FUNDAMENTALISM

This all sounds lovely, you might be thinking, but it's not enough to just share the good news, is it? The passion we're compelled to share when we *become vegan* isn't just about the joy we feel having had an epiphany; it's about the urgency we feel knowing that humans cause the suffering and death of billions of animals every year, or knowing that millions of humans could be saved from preventable diseases and deaths related to the consumption of animal-based saturated fat, cholesterol, and protein. If others were aware of this too, then we could end all this suffering. *That's* the news we need to share, you might say. It's not enough to talk about how great it is to be vegan; we need to talk about how awful it is for the animals destined for human consumption. We need to wake up the public about the institutionalized violence against sentient beings, the systematic destruction of ecosystems, and the devastation we're causing to our own bodies through our insatiable appetite for meat, dairy, and eggs.

This is all true, and later I address how to find your voice (Stage Seven) and how to advocate effectively (Stage Nine). *This* stage, however, is about finding the balance between expressing your passion for being vegan and dictating that others become vegan, because if we don't find this balance, not only will we live in a constant state of dissatisfaction, we will never transcend the public perception about what it means to be vegan—and let's be honest: the public perception of veganism isn't all that positive. In a recent study, 47 percent of all participants felt negatively toward vegetarians and even more so when they felt that vegetarians considered themselves to be morally superior to nonvegetarians.[3] Extrapolate that to vegans, and the percentage is probably even higher. Preachy. Pedantic. Dogmatic. Fanatical. Evangelical. Zealous. Militant. Sanctimonious. Judgmental. Holier-Than-Thou. On Their High Horse. Extremist. Fervent. Fundamentalist. These are just some of the more negative adjectives often used to describe vegans, and though they don't describe *most* vegans, they *are* the stereotype, and sometimes stereotypes are true (otherwise they wouldn't be stereotypes). Notice that our passion is almost never described in less provocative terms. We're not called *enthusiasts, fans,* or *devotees.* The descriptors for vegans are, in fact, the same ones used for religious zealots, and indeed veganism is often likened to a cult.

Strictly speaking, veganism lacks the features commonly seen in organized cults: a single charismatic leader, sexual or economic exploitation of its members, and a methodical process of indoctrination, otherwise called "brainwashing." But literal definitions aside, people do have the perception that:

◆ Veganism consists of a set of rigid rules and doctrines.

◆ Veganism's focus is on ideology and purity.

◆ Vegans "force" their views on others.

◆ Having your own interpretation of veganism is forbidden.

Unfortunately, these perceptions don't come merely from a larger cultural bias against veganism; they come, in part, from vegans—or more accurately, from *vegan fundamentalists.* Although some vegans might bristle at being called *fundamentalist* due to the negative connotations of that word and its association with conservative religious views, just a cursory understanding of *religious fundamentalism* makes the parallels all too apparent.

Fundamentalism in the religious sense refers to a coalition of American Protestants who oppose theological liberalism, modernism, and rationalism and who insist on the infallibility and inerrancy of the Bible. More broadly, in both religious and secular contexts, a fundamentalist is a person who "adheres strictly or dogmatically to the fundamental tenets or principles of any subject, discipline, or movement."[4] Fundamentalism in the general sense is characterized by rigid adherence to certain doctrines, scriptures, ideologies, or principles; intolerance for diversity of opinion; and belief in the "importance of maintaining in-group and out-group distinctions"[5]— with an emphasis on purity and the return to a former ideal.

Looking at the main features of fundamentalism, it's not hard to recognize its presence in the vegan community. (I've generally used Christian fundamentalism here for illustrative purposes, but fundamentalism is prevalent in other religions as well.)

- **Fundamentalists believe in the authority of a written word.** For Christian fundamentalists, it's the Bible in its current form. For vegan fundamentalists, it's *one particular* iteration of the definition of veganism.

- **Fundamentalists believe in the inerrancy of that written word.** For Christian fundamentalists, this means that they believe that every word in the Bible is divinely inspired and cannot be changed or disputed. For vegan fundamentalists, it means that the singular definition of veganism attributed to Vegan Society founder Donald Watson is definitive, authoritative, and incontestable, despite the fact that it was devised and continually revised by various founders and members of the UK Vegan Society from its very beginning and throughout the mid-twentieth century.

- **Fundamentalists rigidly adhere to rules, ideologies, and dogma without question.** For religious fundamentalists, these rules are manifested as doctrines, sacraments, commandments, observances, and laws. For vegan fundamentalists, these rules are manifested in intolerance for exceptions, mistakes, incremental steps, imperfection, or differences in philosophy. People who say they're 99.9 percent vegan are denounced for not being 100 percent vegan, and laws that improve the welfare of farmed animals are condemned (because, fundamentalists would argue, they still condone a system of oppression). Moreover, the very act of *questioning* certain aspects of veganism or acknowledging that there are gray areas is interpreted as being a disloyal or inauthentic vegan.

- **Fundamentalists are intolerant of nuance and diversity of opinion and exile those who don't agree with their perspective.** In both religious and secular fundamentalism, those who don't conform are considered heretics or traitors and are silenced, ostracized, or otherwise punished. In vegan fundamentalism, dialogue is shut down by dismissing perceived dissenters as not being "real" vegans, banning them from online forums, and even shouting down and silencing speakers at public events.

♦ **Fundamentalists believe in the importance of maintaining in-group and out-group distinctions.** Religious fundamentalists dismiss out-groups as infidels. Vegan fundamentalists take moral audits not only of nonvegans (an obvious "out-group") but also of those who self-identify as "plant-based." In other words, even when people abstain from eating animal flesh and fluids, vegan fundamentalists consider them part of the out-group and characterize them as frauds or imposters if they're not doing it "for animals." Justifying the distinction, they cite their own authoritative understanding of the word *vegan*, assert their exclusive claim to the word, and marginalize those who interpret it differently. Conversely, "plant-based fundamentalists" also create in-group and out-group distinctions, dismissing vegans who eat "processed" foods or who don't follow a strict diet of whole foods as "junk-food vegans." The groups get factionalized further still, into "abolitionists" versus "welfarists," for example, or, in the health arena, those who are raw-foodists, WFPB (whole-foods, plant-based), SOS-free (salt/oil/sugar-free), HCLF (high-carb, low-fat), and so on.

♦ **Fundamentalists excommunicate, banish, or shun members as punishment for not adhering to doctrine.** Different religions practice various forms and severity of excommunication—from completely severing someone's ties to the church to allowing them to partake in some aspects while denying them access to others. Vegans can't "kick people out of the club," because there is no homogenous club, but they can deny people legitimacy and identity. Vegan fundamentalists decry the use of the label "vegan" for anyone who doesn't tick all the boxes of what they say *vegan* means, and they call anyone who doesn't submit to their interpretation "fake vegans." It may not be a *literal* excommunication, but it is a kind of *rhetorical* excommunication.

Veganism may not be a religious cult, but it certainly can have the trappings of secular fundamentalism. Or, to be more accurate: when we see veganism as the *goal to attain* rather than as the *means to attaining our goals*, we risk ensnaring ourselves in fundamentalist thinking and behavior. The goal is to live in such a way that doesn't *intentionally* cause harm. The goal is to live according to *compassion* or *wellness*. The goal is not to *live according to veganism*. That would imply that there are rules and doctrines to live by, which is not what being vegan is about. When we think being vegan is the badge to wear or the destination to reach, we treat it as an ideology and obsess over trying to be perfect and pure. If we see veganism as the *goal* rather than as the *means to attain* our goals, not only do we miss the point of what it means to be vegan, we also lead a frustrating existence filled with anger and judgment, and people who might otherwise be interested in using veganism as a tool to reach their own goals (of not hurting animals, of being healthy, of helping the Earth) will be repelled.

The consequences of vegan fundamentalism aren't merely petty online exchanges and virtual chest-beating. They are tribalism, rigidity, close-mindedness, chauvinism, and hostility—all of which distract from the larger goals of protecting animals from harm or of achieving wellness. The average person who stops eating meat, dairy, and eggs isn't looking for a tribal identity; they're just looking to manifest their compassion or eat more healthfully. Labeled as selfish for abstaining from animal products *only* for health

> The goal is to live in such a way that doesn't *intentionally* cause harm. The goal is to live according to *compassion* or *wellness*. The goal is not to *live according to veganism*.

reasons, they're forbidden to call themselves "vegan" by the fundamentalists who guard the word as jealous lovers. Rather than embrace potential allies, fundamentalists reject anyone who fails the impossible litmus test they've devised—and which no one, even them, can pass.

It's a very human impulse to see and be seen in terms of identities, especially those that are important to us, but there are downsides to seeing everything through this lens, including feeling that groups similar to our own undermine the very nature of what makes our group unique. Social psychologists even have a name for this—they call it *categorization threat* or *distinctiveness threat*: when groups too similar to our own threaten the special identity of our group. This may explain why people who self-identify as "ethical vegans" spend so much time criticizing people who stop eating animal products for health reasons. It also may explain why people who self-identify as "plant-based" spend so much time criticizing people they consider "junk-food vegans." These groups may have different underlying goals, but ironically, it's actually the commonalities between them—the choice to stop eating meat, dairy, and eggs—that create the tension. Tobias Leenaert, author of *How to Create a Vegan World*, contemplated this phenomenon on his blog, *The Vegan Strategist*:

> Maybe a club that gets too big is a threat to our identity too. Maybe after a while we are not feeling exclusive or special enough anymore, and that might be why we need to make sure entrance to our in-group doesn't become too easy. The membership fee, in this sense, has to be high enough. The vegan police is there to guard the door.[6]

This connects to what Sigmund Freud called the *narcissism of minor differences*: "the phenomenon that it is precisely communities with adjoining territories and who are related to each other in other ways who are engaged in constant feuds and in ridiculing each other—Germans and South Germans, the English and the Scotch, and so on." In our case: animal welfarists and animal liberationists; "ethical vegans" and "health vegans"; and all the subcategories within. In being obsessed with our minor differences, we lose sight of our major goals.

It's not that we shouldn't have an ideal to aspire to or a code to live by, but when ideology becomes a holy relic to be worshiped rather than an aspiration and a guide, we've lost the plot. When we become more attached to the belief system than to the potential for that belief system to help us accomplish our goals, we've forgotten our purpose. We mistake the finger pointing to the moon for the moon itself.

Remaining engaged but unattached means setting out to inspire rather than setting out to convert. Attracting rather than proselytizing. Being enthusiastic rather than evangelical. So, speak up, speak out, share the good news, be a messenger of compassion, evangelize, and vegangelize! And then . . . let go.

> When ideology becomes a holy relic to be worshiped rather than an aspiration and a guide, we've lost the plot.

Several years ago I received an email from a woman named Christina that perfectly articulates the need to walk that line between speaking your truth and remaining unattached to the outcome:

*I was in the evangelizing stage for a long time when I made the transition to unconditional compassion. I would re-post almost everything I found on the internet about animals. As expected, this just turned people off and probably made a lot of Facebook friends hide my posts. Since then, I have been very careful about what I share. Now, when I post things, I want them to have impact. Recently, an animal protection organization released some footage about wool and lambskin. I already knew about the problems with wool, but I know that many of my friends buy wool often. So, I felt that it was something I needed to share. Instead of just throwing it up on my Facebook page as I had in the past, I made sure to write my own heartfelt message to go along with it. I acknowledged that I need to be careful about what I post online so that I don't overwhelm people but that I felt this was important because wool and lambskin are so popular. I spoke my truth—and stepped back. I actually did not expect to get any responses. I expected the post to be ignored, as past ones had. But it seems that this one actually touched my friends, many of whom left comments about how they had no idea about the treatment of sheep, saying how good it was to be informed. Even my leather-wearing mother, who has mocked my vegan lifestyle, responded saying that she cried while watching the video and reading the article. Even this small thing gives me so much hope. It gives me hope that if we are thoughtful and intentional, we can slowly wake people up to the truth. It takes discipline to speak my truth without following my natural instinct to scold and guilt people, but that just makes them angry and turns them off to the message.*

Indeed, the anger we inspire is the anger we internalize, and it's anger we turn to next. Anger is what follows when our vegan message fails to inspire friends and family to become vegan, when we spread the word about the atrocities committed against animals only to be ignored. The more we encounter resistance and apathy, the more frustrated we feel, and the more strident we become. Anger follows evangelism, because it's at this stage that our own hope begins to wane, when we see the magnitude of the cruelty animals endure, when we feel frustrated that even though we're part of the solution, everyone else is creating the problem.

*Stage Five*

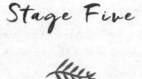

# The Angry Vegan

## *Dispelling the Stereotype and Understanding Its Roots*

Every man has his secret sorrows which the world knows not;
and oftentimes we call a man cold when he is only sad.
—Henry Wadsworth Longfellow

received an email from a young woman several years ago that perfectly illustrates this next stage: anger and disgust on the outside, sorrow and grief on the inside.

*The more I learn about the torture, evil, horrors, and unthinkably cruel acts placed upon our companions, the very ones that (I believe) we are supposed to protect, the more I hurt. I can't stop crying. I can't stop crying for the momma cow following her newborn baby as workers drag him away by a leg. I can't stop crying for the baby piglet picked up then smashed on the floor by a frustrated worker. I can't stop crying for the chicken who is dying because her neck became tangled in a battery cage and she can no longer reach food or water. For the turkeys, goats, sheep, rats, dogs, cats, rabbits, fish, dolphins, seals, bears, and wolves who look at us in their hour of death, fighting until the end. Sometimes I become so angry . . . so angry at my fellow humans and wonder how can we do this? But then I remember that many of us can't even show compassion to our own species and then I cry for them all . . . all the time. As I type I must stop to clear the tears from my eyes. I cry for the lives I cannot save, I cry for the animals who deserve better, I cry for the beings who will never know the natural human capacity to love and my heart aches for the ones who are in my Nebraskan backyard who I cannot protect. I was so excited to be vegan . . . and now I am struggling to cope. Please tell me . . . will the tears ever stop?*

And this one:

*I came across your website and podcast just over two months ago, and I am very thankful that I did. Not only do you speak with compassion, eloquence, and wisdom, you have taught me how to deal with the most difficult situations. Instead of simply being frustrated and intolerant of ignorance, I've implemented your approach to "plant seeds" of change. As a health professional, I really should know that this is the best way to engage with humans, but during many of the months that followed my awakening, all I felt was anger and disgust. I suppose I was grieving, and I was frustrated and angry at myself for my ignorance. All I wanted to do was to make people wake up by sharing my newfound knowledge. I could not understand how they could not be as outraged as I was by the daily atrocities that nonhuman animals endure, but as you know, people need to come around in their own time. I needed to remember that I, too, was disassociated and ignorant not too long ago—and for far too long.*

And another one:

*After seeing a clip online about factory farming, I felt horrible. I immediately stopped eating any dairy or eggs and buying anything taken from an animal (I was already vegetarian). I also obsessively researched and read and watched footage. I saw the unimaginable things that were being done to these beautiful living beings. I was so disgusted and angry, and when I spoke about this with family and friends, no one got it. As accepting as they all were about my vegetarianism, they were very critical about my choice to be vegan.*

And finally:

*After going vegan, I spent a year learning about the horrendous treatment of animals in our society and being angry at the world, unsure of how I would ever fit in it again.*

Not surprisingly, hidden within these stories are all the stages we've already examined:

- "I obsessively researched and read and watched footage." (voracious consumption of information)
- "I spent a year learning about the horrendous treatment of animals in our society." (voracious consumption of information)
- "I was angry at myself for my ignorance." (remorse)
- "When I spoke about this with family and friends, no one got it." (coming out)
- "All I wanted to do was to make people wake up by sharing my newfound knowledge." (evangelism)

Common threads run through the story of every vegan I've ever heard from or spoken to, especially vegans who make the change for ethical reasons; there is anger, sorrow, grief, disenchantment, and despair in almost all of them. This stage is particularly tricky, because the awareness that may have compelled us to make a change in the first place is the very same awareness that can weigh us down—and keep us down. This stage is familiar to most vegans, and although entering it might be inevitable, remaining stuck in it is not. Of course anger is only one aspect of what we feel once we become vegan, and peace is one of the byproducts of living a compassionate life. Many new and veteran vegans describe feeling a profound sense of relief and a deep peace of mind as the result of living in harmony with their values. But, whereas stopping our participation in the institutionalized exploitation of other animals does bring peace of mind, the awareness of so much cruelty and suffering can also have a devastating effect on our psyches. Burnout is common among vegans and animal advocates, and many become jaded, hopeless, self-righteous, and angry.

And why shouldn't we be angry? Human greed and the desire for convenience and pleasure drive the socially sanctioned use and abuse of billions of nonhuman animals. We live in a world where it's considered normal to champion this and radical to oppose it. Of course we are angry. But anger is not a dirty word, and to remain a vegan—and a joyful one, in particular—is to understand its roots, which are planted in sorrow and anguish. The earliest meaning of the word *anger* reflects this: it referred to something being "painfully constricted"—a strangling, a narrowing, a squeezing, a throttling—and our modern word *anger* comes from an Old Norse word meaning *anguish*. If we reframe anger to see it in its historical context, we recognize that there isn't a contradiction between the peace that comes with eating nonviolently and the anger we feel in the face of so much cruelty. In other words, while we may experience anger on the surface, something much more tender is underneath—and I believe that something is *sorrow*.

In all the years I've been listening to people's experiences, as well as tapping into my own, I've come to believe that *sorrow* is at the core of our emotional reaction to the injustices imposed on animals—but *anger* is just easier to manifest. It's familiar, it's recognizable, and it's culturally supported. Anger has gravitas. Sorrow and sadness are interpreted as weak and ineffectual; some people, especially men, may even feel ashamed to show sadness at all, since vulnerability implies frailty in a culture that values masculine traits. I hear from both men and women who tell me they don't know how to talk about animal issues without crying or demonstrating sadness—as if showing such emotions would negate or undermine the seriousness of their message and beliefs. And so either they say nothing at all or they display the more socially acceptable emotion of anger, which—ironically—can have deleterious effects on their message, on their relationships, and on themselves.

Anger is a natural human emotion and certainly shouldn't be ignored or suppressed, but depending on its frequency, duration, and intensity, anger can be detrimental to our mental, emotional, and physical health. The stress hormones triggered by anger contribute to the fight-or-flight response that protects us from danger; a constant flood of these chemicals and their associated metabolic changes, however, can also strain our cardiovascular, immune, digestive, and central nervous systems. Anger causes an elevated heart rate, increased blood pressure, and high blood glucose levels, which can lead to stroke or heart attack.[1] Another side effect of anger, decreased blood flow, can lead to digestive issues, headaches, migraines, and insomnia. Even a short burst of anger can impair the immune system for several hours after,[2] and, if sustained, can lead to an increased risk of infection, and possibly even cancer.[3] Chronic anger is linked to unhappiness, low self-esteem, self-harm, drug and alcohol addiction, depression, poor peer relationships, and a greater likelihood of abusing others physically or mentally.[4]

Self-compassion should be reason enough to be wary of chronic anger, but many vegans and animal advocates cling to it as fuel. A popular axiom circulating in many social justice–oriented circles—not just among vegans—says that *if you're not outraged, you're not paying attention.*

Moral indignation becomes a measure of how much we care. If we're not cynical about the past and pessimistic about the future, then we're apathetic, delusional, or willfully ignoring injustice and violence. The world becomes a zero-sum game of offenders and defenders, victims and warriors, sinners and saints. The entire human population becomes an enemy to defeat, a scourge to extinguish. Operating within this framework, it's no surprise, then, that well-intentioned advocates tell themselves that to let go of anger implies that they're choosing inertia and inaction; letting go of anger becomes tantamount to betraying the animals who desperately need our intervention. The anger that would be a *means* for change becomes the *end* in itself, and being an angry vegan becomes a point of pride, a mark of identity characterized by misanthropy and disgust. What may have been someone's primary motivating force for change—both their own personal change as well as the change they wish to bring about in the world—becomes the destination. As a result, many become addicted to outrage and mistake it for activism.

> Many become addicted to outrage and mistake it for activism.

The problems with this model are manifold: not only does sustained anger not feel good, it's also not effective or productive. People are always looking for ways to dismiss vegans as radical and animal advocates as crazy, and nothing gives them more opportunity to do so than the presence of the angry vegan. People simply don't respond well to anger and outrage, which tend to manifest themselves as self-righteousness, martyrdom, indignation, and judgment—all of which corrupt intelligent discourse and turn people off or make them defensive. Not only is prolonged outrage ruinous on one's state of being, it's simply not sustainable, which is why the angriest activists are the first ones to burn out. Our anger may be justified, and indignation may make us feel virtuous, but neither changes hearts, minds, or laws on behalf of animals.

Fortunately, it's not a zero-sum game. We can be passionate, powerful, and productive without being misanthropic or self-destructive. We can be acutely aware, actively engaged, and happier and more effective as a result. We can decide at any given moment whether we want to be an angry vegan or a joyful vegan; the choice is ours. Choosing to lead rather than react, inspire rather than agitate, and guide rather than goad are just a few examples of subtle ways we can direct our passion without losing our purpose. (See the sidebar on page 160 for more.)

> We can be passionate, powerful, and productive without being misanthropic or self-destructive. We can be acutely aware, actively engaged, and happier and more effective as a result.

Joyful vegans aren't perfect, and they certainly aren't saints. They don't think they're better than anyone else; they just know they're better than they were before they *became vegan.* They see veganism as a manifestation of and means to reflect their highest values rather than as an end in itself, and they aspire to act from integrity and compassion—behind closed doors and in public, online and in person, with vegans and with nonvegans. The joyful vegan has no less determination to end violence against animals than the angry vegan, but she is more willing to find resolution than she is eager to be right; she is more interested in solving the problem than she is determined to claim the moral high-ground.

As I've reiterated a couple of times already, these stages are descriptive rather than prescriptive; I'm not suggesting that you should *choose* to be angry if it's not how you feel. If you've never experienced anger in the context I've discussed, that's great. I'm also not suggesting that you try to avoid or deny anger if that is what you feel. But I am cautioning against allowing yourself to inhabit *chronic* anger and treating anger as an end rather than a means.

## HOW TO BE A JOYFUL VEGAN

So, how do you go from being an angry vegan to a joyful vegan—or at least move in that direction? I think the first step is owning that you may need to spend a little time mourning the loss of who you once were, the ignorance you once enjoyed, and the feeling of innocence you once had before you became awake. The next step is embracing and expressing the anguish and the sorrow that underpin the anger you may be feeling in the face of that awakening. As I mentioned above, I hear from many people who want to talk to others about animal issues, but when they try to, they just break down and cry. And so out of the desire to be stalwart ambassadors, they suppress their feelings and their tears, hindering their emotional, mental, and physical well-being in the process. My advice: *cry*. Yes, even while you're talking to others. Of course, there are appropriate and inappropriate times to cry, but exhibiting *emotion* when talking about an *emotional* issue is not only healing (our bodies produce a morphine-like painkiller called leucine enkephalin when we cry), it may very well make us better spokespeople for animals. Evolutionary biologists found that tears may actually make interpersonal relationships stronger. "Crying is a highly evolved behavior," explains evolutionary biologist Oren Hasson of Tel Aviv University. "Tears can elicit mercy from an antagonistic enemy and . . . enhance attachments and friendships."[5] I'm not suggesting we break down sobbing whenever we talk about animal suffering, but I am suggesting that we not be afraid if our voice shakes or our eyes well up. Hasson's findings suggest that tears can inspire sympathy and even strategic assistance, which is why sadness is more effective than anger when talking to people about animal issues. I don't think we should have the expectation that people *will* respond more sympathetically, but there is no doubt they will respond more positively to vulnerability than to a wall of anger.

The next step in transcending anger is related to something we discussed back in chapter one on the voracious consumption of information: we have to be honest with ourselves about how much suffering we can endure to witness. That might mean avoiding looking at images, watching documentaries, or reading stories that depict violence against animals—at least for a while. It may mean not attending vigils—a relatively new, popular form of activism whereby a group of people bear witness to animals being trucked to slaughter (and sometimes intervene by giving them water). Of course bearing witness is necessary and noble, but it doesn't mean we have to do it all the time. Just because we look doesn't mean we have to stare. Some vegans feel they are letting animals down if they don't perpetually dwell on how bad it is for them—if they don't take on the same suffering as the animals. That's not advocacy; that's martyrdom. And it's not effective; it's self-indulgent—and potentially self-destructive. The risks of immersing ourselves in animal cruelty are very high, potentially leading to depression, chronic anger, empathic distress, and even apathy. Self-preservation isn't selfish. It's imperative. Animals don't need us to be as distressed as they are. They need us to transcend our distress so that we can successfully end theirs.

Anger and outrage are both cultivated. You have to work to keep them alive. If all we focus on is violence, cruelty, and abuse, we convince ourselves there is nothing else. There is indeed misery and suffering in the world, but that's not *all* there is. At any given moment, we can choose to focus on one truth or another, and in doing so form our worldview. We become what we focus on, because we *are* our thoughts. Don't underestimate the power of thought; it shapes our perceptions, it determines our actions, and it creates the world we envision. If we believe that cruelty and injustice will prevail, then that's what we will manifest. If we believe that justice and compassion will prevail, that's what we will ensure. In any given moment, we can choose despair and anger, or we can choose compassion and hope.

> Animals don't need us to be as distressed as they are. They need us to transcend our distress so that we can successfully end theirs.

I choose hope—my third prescription for transforming anger.

I honestly could not do this work or call myself a joyful vegan if I did not have hope—or rather, if I did not choose to *dwell* in hope—and no, my hope is neither delusional nor naïve. It is rooted in facts, science, reason, and statistics. I have hope because there's much to be hopeful about. History gives you great perspective if you just step back. My hope is not complacent; it's provisional. I don't just sit back and want things to change; I take action to facilitate that change because I believe change can happen; I dwell on what I can solve rather than on what I can't. There are plenty of reasons to be angry at the injustices in the world—there always will be—but there are plenty of reasons to be hopeful because of progress in the world, too. We can decide which we want to focus on, and I choose the latter. I have hope because I choose to. Like anger, hope is also cultivated. You have to work at it to keep it alive.

A fourth way to transform anger into joy is through laughter, which I indulge in every day. Although I do tend to consume books and films of a darker nature, when my husband and I sit down after a long day, we always make a point to watch some of our favorite comedy shows or stand-up comics, some of which we've seen multiple times but which never fail to deliver. Humor is incredibly healing, and it is a mandatory prescription for transcending anger. Scientifically proven to benefit our mental and physical health, laughter relieves tension, boosts energy, increases resilience, releases endorphins, reduces stress, reinforces social connections, strengthens the immune system, counteracts feelings of anxiety and sadness, and—simply and unsurprisingly—reduces anger and increases joy. Find your favorite sources of laughter, and luxuriate in it.

My fifth suggestion for alleviating anger (while still remaining engaged) is to connect with others. Being part of a community is vital for us as social creatures, and while having like-minded people in our life helps us feel less alone and part of a united front (see the next stage, Finding Your Tribe), we need to also feel accepted and loved within that community. Being connected also means feeling that you're part of your larger society—and even your species! After all, how can you transform something you disengage from? Being connected means resisting the "us versus them" mentality—which I address at length in Stage Seven and which can be healed using the Loving-Kindness Meditation on page 81.

In addition to connecting with others, laughing, dwelling in hope rather than despair, and allowing yourself to cry, there are many other strategies for transcending negative emotions:

- → Create a mindfulness practice.
- → Meditate.
- → Keep a journal.
- → Learn relaxation and breathing techniques.
- → Consult a therapist.
- → Devise a self-care plan that includes eating well and exercising.

Remember: outrage doesn't change the world. Vision and vigilance do—along with the political, technological, economic, and moral forces that drive progress forward. We don't have to be angry all the time to demonstrate we care. We don't have to be outraged to show that we're conscious. We can develop what Buddhist teacher and Zen priest Joan Halifax calls strong back/soft front: "Instead of having a strong back, many of us have a defended front shielding a weak spine . . . and we walk around brittle and defensive. If we strengthen our backs, metaphorically speaking, and develop a spine that's flexible but sturdy, then we can risk having a front that's soft and open. It is the strong back that supports the soft front of compassion."[6]

> Outrage doesn't change the world. Vision and vigilance do.

## Traits of an Angry Vegan Versus a Joyful Vegan

Although I've been talking about the detrimental effects of being an angry vegan for decades, I'm not the only one. Fellow writer and advocate Andrew Kirschner has a blog called *Kirschner's Korner*, which is filled with insightful, compassionate commentary about vegans and vegan advocates, including one post called "The Angry Vegan," which inspired the distinctions I've created below.

The angry vegan condemns. *The joyful vegan supports.*

The angry vegan judges. *The joyful vegan analyzes.*

The angry vegan rants. *The joyful vegan informs.*

The angry vegan raves. *The joyful vegan articulates.*

The angry vegan criticizes. *The joyful vegan discerns.*

The angry vegan demands. *The joyful vegan entreats.*

The angry vegan shouts. *The joyful vegan communicates.*

The angry vegan vilifies. *The joyful vegan commends.*

The angry vegan antagonizes. *The joyful vegan attracts.*

The angry vegan reacts. *The joyful vegan leads.*

The angry vegan silences. *The joyful vegan listens.*

The angry vegan agitates. *The joyful vegan inspires.*

The angry vegan provides shock. *The joyful vegan provokes thought.*

The angry vegan polices language. *The joyful vegan masters language.*

The angry vegan enrages the public. *The joyful vegan engages the public.*

The angry vegan goads. *The joyful vegan guides.*

The angry vegan polarizes. *The joyful vegan unites.*

The angry vegan scowls. *The joyful vegan smiles.*

The angry vegan insults. *The joyful vegan influences.*

The angry vegan guilts. *The joyful vegan directs.*

The angry vegan alienates. *The joyful vegan motivates.*

The angry vegan forces. *The joyful vegan encourages.*

The angry vegan intimidates. *The joyful vegan persuades.*

The angry vegan sees only problems. *The joyful vegan finds solutions.*

The angry vegan makes enemies. *The joyful vegan makes allies.*

The angry vegan expels dissenters. *The joyful vegan welcomes ideas.*

The angry vegan is impatient. *The joyful vegan is earnest.*

The angry vegan is inflexible. *The joyful vegan is adaptable.*

The angry vegan is intolerant. *The joyful vegan is understanding.*

The angry vegan is rigid. *The joyful vegan is supple.*

The angry vegan is combative. *The joyful vegan is provocative.*

The angry vegan is irascible. *The joyful vegan is passionate.*

The angry vegan is impolitic. *The joyful vegan is diplomatic.*

The angry vegan is dogmatic. *The joyful vegan is outspoken.*

The angry vegan is arrogant. *The joyful vegan is receptive.*

The angry vegan is ideological. *The joyful vegan is visionary.*

The angry vegan is pessimistic. *The joyful vegan is hopeful.*

The angry vegan sees only one path. *The joyful vegan sees many.*

The angry vegan speaks condescendingly. *The joyful vegan speaks respectfully.*

The angry vegan finds fault with imperfections. *The joyful vegan knows that being vegan means being imperfect, because vegans are human.*

The angry vegan sees evil. *The joyful vegan sees fear.*

The angry vegan cares nothing for public opinion. *The joyful vegan values her role as a public ambassador.*

The angry vegan forgets he once ate animal products. *The joyful vegan remembers.*

The angry vegan demands compassion for nonhuman animals while excoriating human animals. *The joyful vegan strives to have compassion for everyone, even for those who are not compassionate.*

The angry vegan says, "Do everything" to aspiring vegans. *The joyful vegan says, "Don't do nothing."*

# Finding Your Tribe

## *Embracing Your Identity, Building Community, and Feeling a Sense of Belonging*

No man is an island, entire of itself. Any man's death diminishes
me, because I am involved in mankind; and therefore never
send to know for whom the bell tolls; it tolls for thee.

—John Donne

S ocial creatures through and through, humans yearn to be part
of a community of like-minded people who share similar goals,
interests, and values. Psychologist Abraham Maslow placed social
belonging just after basic physiological and safety needs in his hierarchy

of needs, first posited in 1943. According to Maslow, meeting basic needs such as hunger, thirst, safety, and security comes first, but belong-ingness immediately follows, taking precedence over self-esteem, self-actualization, and self-transcendence. Researchers who both preceded and followed Maslow asserted similar *need-to-belong* theories but with more of an emphasis on sexual drives and parental bonds and attach-ments. It wasn't until 1995 that social psychologists Roy Baumeister and Mark Leary empirically demonstrated that humans are *fundamentally* driven by the need to belong to and be valued by social groups and that this need is strongly rooted in our evolutionary history. Providing survival and reproductive benefits, as well as emotional, cognitive, and physical ones, our need to belong, they argue, "can be almost as compelling a need as food." In other words, humans have survived and thrived over these millennia because of our bonds with one another.

As social animals, we evolved in small communal groups that relied on close alliances—sharing mutual goals, working together to achieve common objectives, and protecting one another from various threats. Cooperation benefited everyone in the tribe, but it also strengthened bonds, and even enhanced feelings of self-worth and esteem. "Evidence suggests," write Baumeister and Leary, "that being accepted, included, or welcomed leads to a variety of positive emotions (e.g., happiness, ela-tion, contentment, and calm)." The inverse is also true: Considerable research shows that *not* having a sense of belonging leaves people sus-ceptible to loneliness, social anxiety, mental distress, and clinical depres-sion.[1] A study by Naomi Eisenberger, a social psychologist and director of the Social and Affective Neuroscience Laboratory at UCLA, revealed that "the same neurochemicals that regulate physical pain also control the psychological pain of social loss."[2] When we connect with others, it stimulates the production of opioids, which makes us feel really good. On the flip side, when social connections break down and relationships disintegrate, opioids are not produced, and we feel bad. In short, lack of acceptance among social groups triggers emotional distress. Our need to belong to a community—large or small—is as great as our need for air or water; without it, we fail to thrive.

When it comes to becoming and staying vegan, this is where the rubber meets the road. According to the research, feelings of social isolation and pressure from one's peers and family members can be the hardest part of living a vegan lifestyle. In Faunalytics' study of lapsed vegetarians and vegans, 63 percent of former vegetarians/vegans said that they didn't like how it made them stick out from the crowd, and almost half said they didn't have sufficient interactions with fellow vegans or vegetarians. And 84 percent of those who reverted to eating animals reported that they were not active in vegetarian or vegan clubs or organizations.[3]

These data suggest that the need to belong is so strong that many people would rather be disconnected from their own values than be disconnected from other people. In social science studies that examine why it's so hard to change behavior we know is causing harm, the conclusions continually point toward the fact that "social norms constrain human behavior, as the mere thought of doing something drastically different from what others are doing, or what others appear to approve of, can lead to intense feelings of discomfort, embarrassment, or shame."[4]

> The need to belong is so strong that many people would rather be disconnected from their own values than be disconnected from other people.

Here is a letter from a podcast listener named Jesse that I think represents thousands of other, unwritten letters.

*After going vegan, I spent a year learning about the horrendous treatment of animals in our society and being angry at the world, unsure of how I would ever fit in again. Oddly enough, as passionate as I was about not contributing to animal suffering ever again, I fell off the wagon a year later and reverted to eating (and even wearing) animal products. I now realize this was largely due to having felt completely alone, isolated, and hopeless. I was the only vegan I knew at the time, and what support I had from nonvegan friends and family was superficial at best; at times I was ridiculed and criticized for eschewing animal products. I felt like I was the only one trying to do the right thing and ultimately gave up! Some months later, I thankfully got myself back on track, but I knew that I would not be able to stay vegan without some kind of support.*

Jesse's story is a testament to the fact that awareness, passion, and compassion aren't always enough to stay vegan. Aside from the fact that she was probably deep in empathic distress (see Stage One) and clearly suffering from hopelessness and unresolved anger (see Stage Five), she was also living in a kind of no-man's-land that so many find themselves in—feeling disconnected from nonvegan friends and family while belonging to no tribe that speaks their language. But the distress that Jesse and so many like her feel doesn't only come from lacking like-minded people they can relate to, or from feeling detached from those they love; it also comes from the pressure to conform to the values and gastronomic habits of their friends, family, and culture—and dealing with disappointment or criticism when they don't. This is exactly what happened to podcast listener Stacey:

*I am a returning vegan. I was vegan a few years ago for approximately two years for health and weight reasons but reverted back due to lack of support from family and friends. The teasing and rudeness got worse with time, and I wasn't educated enough to make much of an argument in defense of veganism. I switched back to meat eating for a year, but it never felt right to me. This year, I began to actually feel sick to my stomach and sick to my heart if I ate meat. I knew I was becoming more conscious of the animals I was putting in my mouth, and over time it became more about them than about me. So, I took the time and effort to start over. This time, applying your suggestions for overcoming the social challenges, I am now a compassionate, joyful vegan.*

Luckily for them and the animals, both Jesse and Stacey realized they needed to boost their social support in order to stay vegan the second time around, but it goes to show that as much as we want to avoid causing harm to animals, competing motives such as the need to belong and the desire to fit in play equally strong roles in determining our behavior. The price for group membership often involves conforming to the norms of others, and when it comes to what we eat, there is perhaps no greater socially accepted norm than the consumption of animal-based meat, milk, and eggs. "Most people eat meat because most people eat meat,"[5] as advocate and vegan strategist Tobias Leenaert observes. So, despite our own ethics or health concerns or whatever compels us to stop eating animal flesh and fluids, we may continue to do so for fear of being different. Or we may stop being vegan because the social pressure to eat animal products is simply too great. And the key to combating both of those is celebrating all aspects of who we are and how we identify.

## EMBRACING OUR IDENTITIES

The desire to belong is both a barrier to entry for meat-eaters and a cause for recidivism among vegetarians and vegans. We often hear that individuality is valued in our culture—and of course it is—but we have enough empirical data and anecdotal evidence to conclude that we value conformity a lot more. *Nonconformist* is a dirty word in many people's vocabulary, and the consequences of dissenting can be severe—namely becoming a persona non grata and being cast out from our group (and even from more than one group). It may not be a literal exile, but it can certainly feel that way, as our need to belong plays out in both subtle and direct ways. Our fear of not pleasing everyone around us can paralyze us and compel us to favor someone else's desire for us to conform over our own desire to do what we feel is right. A recent article reviewing how humans respond to environmental crises grappled with this very dilemma: "Psychologists do not yet know why some [people] are willing or able to take a bold stand for change in the same situations that drive others to support the status quo or to simply withdraw. What they do know is that resisting the pressure to conform . . . requires nothing short of heroic effort."[6]

There's an ancient Arabic folktale about a witch who visits a kingdom one night and taints the public well with a poison that drives people mad. The next morning, all the villagers drink the water and indeed go mad. The king avoids drinking the well water and thus remains sane. Later that same day, the villagers arrive at the king's palace and accuse *him* of being mad. The king realizes he has a decision to make. He could drink from the well, lose his sanity, and conform to everyone else in his kingdom, while remaining king. Or he could *not* drink, and remain sane, but be deposed from his throne by those who see his sanity as madness. For ordinary folk like you and me, the stakes may not be as high as those in this story, but I think they feel that way to many of us. Though we may not have a kingdom to lose, we're often afraid of losing relationships or even just our own sense of comfort, and these things are as valuable to an ordinary citizen as a kingdom is to a king.

Because our veganism may be seen as antithetical to the other communities to which we belong, we may as a result become less liked, perceived as suspicious, or considered deviant. Similar to reactions we received when we *came out vegan*:

- We may be accused of rejecting our cultural heritage: "This is the way our family has eaten for generations. It's part of our culture."
- We may be accused of turning our back on our family lineage and thus insulting individual members: "How can you do this to your grandmother? It would break her heart if you didn't eat her [fill-in-the-blank] dish on Thanksgiving."
- Our choice is taken as a personal affront: "You've always loved what I cook for you, and now suddenly it's not good enough? How can you be so ungrateful?"

- We're told to fend for ourselves: "I'm not going to the fuss of making a separate meal for you. If you want to eat this way, you're on your own."

We're even accused of denying our evolutionary heritage as human beings. The argument goes something like this: Since early humans ate animals, we're justified in continuing to eat them now. And so it follows that vegans—in eschewing animal flesh and fluids—are turning their backs on their evolutionary heritage and sacrificing a part of their human identity. Surely, our identities are defined by more than our paleontological past. Besides, do we really want to use Neanderthals as the model for our ethics? Can't we do better than that? We often say that we want to do better than we did a generation ago, two generations ago—I presume we also want to do better than we did tens or hundreds of thousands of years ago. Isn't that the point of being human—to learn from our past and make better, more healthful, more compassionate choices once we know better and have the ability and opportunity to do so?

It's not only our place in the group that can become questioned and even threatened when we become vegan; it's our own individual identity. A large number of people resist labeling themselves "vegan"—even if they tick all the boxes of what "vegan" means. There are a multitude of reasons for this, and for some people, all of them apply:

- They want to avoid the negative stereotypes associated with the word.
- They eat only whole, raw plant foods and associate "vegan" with highly processed foods.
- They don't want their personal choices to undergo public scrutiny.
- They want the flexibility to occasionally consume animal products.
- They just want to eat without being interrogated.
- They are afraid of "not doing it right" and therefore looking like a failure or a hypocrite.

- They are afraid of being judged for being imperfect (and they associate being vegan with perfectionism).
- They don't want to be accused of being a fake or a fraud by fundamentalist vegans.

But one of the key reasons people choose not to describe themselves as vegan is that they don't want to take on "vegan" as an identity. In fact, in Faunalytics' study of lapsed and current vegetarians and vegans, 58 percent of former vegetarians/vegans said they never saw vegetarianism/veganism as part of their identity, which may be one explanation for their recidivism. In contrast, 89 percent of current vegetarians/vegans did see vegetarianism/veganism as part of their identity.[7] This doesn't mean that in order to stay vegan you have to call yourself "vegan," but it may mean shifting your perception to see *not eating animal products* as more about who you are than just about what you do. Research shows that we tend to place more value on something that is part of our identity; it's the difference between "I *am* vegan" and "I *eat* vegan" or between "I *am* plant-based" and "I *eat* plant-based."

Because our identity is relative to the social groups to which we belong, when we feel isolated from these groups, it can rock us to our core, altering how we see ourselves and how we relate to others. When our existing identity, rooted in family, culture, religion, politics, and/or gender, collides with our vegan identity, we experience a great deal of conflict—both interpersonal and intrapersonal—and may feel compelled to choose one over the other. This conflict often serves as a justification for making no change at all or for returning to eating meat, dairy, or eggs: "My background is German; I could never be vegan." "I come from Irish stock; my meat-and-potatoes family just couldn't take it." "My Jewish grandmother would roll over in her grave if I stopped eating chopped liver!" "I'm a Texan; BBQ is in our bones!" In other words, we often hear that being vegan is incongruent with being . . . well, name it. There isn't one cultural group I haven't heard cited as one whose food traditions are antithetical to veganism. Here are excerpts from a few letters I've received over the years regarding national identity and food traditions:

"Here in Brazil there is a really strong culture around barbecue, and it makes being vegan difficult."

"I'm from Uruguay, and no one understands why I want options that don't include meat, dairy, or eggs."

"Here in Sweden, cheese, dairy, and meat are a part of everything, so just talking about the concept of 'veganism' has been really difficult."

"I live in Denmark, which probably has the world's highest intake of meat per inhabitant. Even being a vegetarian here is considered extreme."

"Because Mongolia is a heavy meat-eating country, I'm often told that it's not suitable for a Mongolian to abstain from meat. Everyone around me says it's simply not *the Mongolian way*."

"It's sacrilege to be vegetarian here in Argentina."

"New Zealand is entrenched in animal agriculture, so much so that milk and whey are in everything."

"Being in Colombia, I find that it is not very friendly to plant-based eating. There are a lot of cultural biases toward eating meat."

"I'm in the UK, where vegan food isn't as readily available as it is in the US."

Do you see what I'm getting at? Most cultures have a history of heavy meat and/or dairy consumption; there are few that don't, particularly as they became wealthier and more industrialized. Food is indeed a significant expression of culture, and we become very attached to the foods we grew up with and the recipes that have been handed down to us, but there are questions we have to ask ourselves:

"Is my cultural heritage reason enough to *not* make some modifications that are in alignment with my current values?"

"Are there other ways—including through food—that I can express and preserve the traditions of my ancestors while still honoring my desire to be vegan?"

Meat, dairy, and eggs are indeed prevalent in many cuisines, but so are plant foods. With a vegan's-eye view of the world, we can just as easily and legitimately celebrate our family history and cultural traditions through the vegetables, fruits, grains, beans, lentils, fungi, herbs, and spices that characterize the cuisine of our heritage—whatever that heritage might be. For instance, here are some examples:

- Maize has provided daily sustenance to Mexicans ever since it was domesticated by the indigenous people of Mexico over ten thousand years ago. Throughout this vast region and across all socioeconomic classes, maize remains the foundation of Mexican cuisine, enjoyed in a variety of forms, from food (tortillas, tamales, tacos) to beverages (atole, champurrado, pozol). In addition to maize, beans, amaranth, and chia were the main crops of Aztec cultures and were even considered suitable as tributes to the gods. Other foods the Mesoamerican people regularly ate that the rest of the world now enjoys are tomatoes, avocados, squash, vanilla, and chocolate. That's a lot to celebrate.

- Soybeans and tea remain staples in Chinese cuisine, which greatly influenced the Japanese, who added them (in the form of miso, tofu, and shoyu) to their repertoire of seaweed, rice, noodles (udon and soba), and vegetables. Mushrooms are also prevalent in Asian cuisines.

- Southern Asian dishes feature a variety of vegetables and aromatic herbs and spices, inspiring many types of curries and broths. Indeed, in many regions of India, vegetarianism is the norm.

♦ Comprising a large variety of countries and peoples, Middle Eastern and Mediterranean cuisines boast hundreds of commonly consumed and highly regarded plant-based ingredients, including olives, olive oil, pistachios, sesame seeds, dates, figs, pomegranates, eggplants, legumes (particularly fava beans and chickpeas), lentils, and a variety of deep-flavored herbs and spices such as coriander, cinnamon, turmeric, saffron, and garlic. First cultivated in the regions of the Fertile Crescent around ten thousand years ago, wheat constitutes the foundation of many Middle Eastern dishes in the form of breads, bulgur, and couscous. Who could say you're turning your back on your Middle Eastern roots when you center your diet on dolmas, falafel, hummus, baba ghanoush, tabbouleh—and coffee?

Instead of seeing the consumption of plant foods as a rejection of our cultural communities, we can see it as a celebration—simply shifting our emphasis away from one type of traditional food and over to another.

But no matter how much we romanticize the notion of cultural tradition, the truth is our attachment to it is not as tenacious as we make it out to be. Throughout our lives, we selectively choose which customs and traditions we want to uphold depending on how convenient, healthful, or ethical they are. We take what we want from the past to create our myths, customs, and traditions, and we leave behind what doesn't suit us anymore. We change our ancestors' recipes based on which ingredients are available or what our family's taste preferences dictate. We modify our relatives' recipes to make them healthier or hypoallergenic. (They most likely made several changes of their own

> Instead of seeing the consumption of plant foods as a rejection of our cultural communities, we can see it as a celebration.

before handing them down to us.) We don't have to perfectly replicate a recipe to honor its creator; it's not only impractical, it's impossible. Brands disappear, vegetables and fruits are modified, tastes change, kitchen tools are improved. The idea is to celebrate the spirit of our traditions rather than create perfect reproductions of them. We turn to cultural customs and family heirlooms because they act as bridges to the past; our desire to feel connected to something older and greater than ourselves is really what we value.

The same is true regarding our religious identity:

"I'm Jewish/Christian/Muslim/Pagan; therefore, I'm compelled/expected to consume meat/dairy/eggs."

Just as with our cultural customs, we pick and choose which aspects of religious texts and tenets we want to follow in our everyday lives to suit our modern tastes and desires. When it comes to the consumption of meat, dairy, and eggs—or abstention from them—messages have varied and rules have been relaxed again and again throughout the centuries, depending on how certain scriptures have been interpreted or translated, on what types of meat were available or affordable (and to whom), on socioeconomic factors, on cultural preferences, on climate, class, and convenience. In other words, in all world religions, we can just as easily find support for eating plant foods as we can justifications for consuming meat and other animal products. Here, too, it's a matter of what we focus on.

Plant foods with symbolic meanings abound in many religions. And yet because the majority of the members in religious communities eat animal flesh and fluids (save for a few holidays where they're asked to abstain for a short period of time), it's the animal products that vegetarians and vegans *don't* eat that people use as evidence that they are snubbing their religious community and upbringing, As a result, vegans can feel detached from yet another group to which they may have once felt a connection, and the pressure to conform may eventually outweigh the desire to do the right thing for themselves, the Earth, or the animals.

It doesn't have to be that way. The foods and rituals associated with religious holidays and observances are really *symbols* for something much deeper, and in being attached to the *form* (eggs at Easter, lamb shank at Passover, for instance), we risk losing the true meaning of whatever it is we are celebrating or honoring. If we uncover the meanings of these symbols, we even find that a plant-based menu better reflects the values and significance of these holidays—renewal and rebirth at Easter, freedom and mercy at Passover—and we can celebrate with foods that are more congruent with those values—namely spring vegetables and matzoh, respectively. These plant foods are already a significant part of these holidays; there's no reason they can't take center stage. Just because the animal products are absent doesn't mean the meaning behind the holiday or religious observance is.

In addition to cultural and religious identity, gender identity is another area that often collides with the vegan identity. Although we're seeing evidence of it shifting, the cultural association between meat and masculinity is deep and persistent. According to a recent survey by the UK's Vegan Society and *Vegan Life* magazine, 63 percent of respondents who identified as vegan were female, while only 37 percent were male.[8] The ratio is similar in the United States. "Meat remains for many men a stable, if arbitrary, hook on which to hang their gender identity," says sociologist Richard Twine, and that has huge implications for men's behavioral choices as well as their standing in the larger community. A year-long research project by scientists from the University of Southampton found that the men in the study experienced "social isolation" after admitting to friends that they were reducing their consumption of meat. Their social shame was so great that—even if they didn't like meat or were directed by their doctors to eat less of it for medical reasons—they had difficulty ordering the vegetarian or vegan option at restaurants for fear of being ridiculed.[9]

Results from numerous studies[10] confirm the strong connection in the public's mind between eating meat—especially muscle meat, like steak—and being masculine. Meat is considered manly; plant foods are considered effeminate. Meat connotes virility; plant foods, effeminacy. In surveys, vegetarians are considered virtuous but also less masculine—as if we can be only one or the other. The media and those in the business of selling animal flesh reinforce the tropes about masculinity and meat with tired stereotypes and offensive ads that claim that meat is manly and tofu is for wimps. *Real men eat meat*, so the marketing slogan goes.

At this point, I know I'm supposed to counter the image of the stereotype by pointing to all the vegan bodybuilders and endurance athletes who are beautifully demonstrating that you don't need to eat meat and other animal products to be strong, fast, and muscular. Though that's true, I'm reluctant to perpetuate such a narrow view of masculinity. Although I'm thrilled there are vegan men demonstrating to themselves and others that you can build muscle and win Ironman competitions fueled by plants, that's still only one facet of masculinity. Having strength isn't measured only by the number of pounds you can lift; it's also about standing firm in your principles, having the courage of your convictions, and exerting control over your own behavior and destiny. Responsibility, integrity, consistency, discipline, logic, being protective, being a good provider—all of these are traditional masculine attributes to be proud of, and none of them are antithetical to being vegan, as this letter from a male podcast listener attests to:

> As a heterosexual twenty-six-year-old guy I could really relate to the content in your podcast episode about how a lot of men believe that eating and cooking meat is "manly." Unfortunately I think that this belief is keeping a lot of men from becoming vegan. I know, for myself, before I became vegan, I had some insecurity about how veganism would affect my masculinity. The only vegans I knew at the time were women and homosexual men, and with all the societal propaganda equating meat eating to masculinity, it was easy to have doubts. I've been vegan for eleven months now and am happy to announce that so far veganism has affected my masculinity in a very positive way. I feel physically healthier, stronger, and I have more energy. I

*also feel more confident in social settings because I have become comfortable doing what I think is right without the need to conform to social norms.*

The association between meat and masculinity affects women as well. If meat makes the man, then the woman who feeds him vegetables is emasculating him. I've lost count of the number of times in the last twenty years my husband was asked if he would still be vegan if I weren't around. The implication is that I *made* David vegan, that I've "whipped" him into giving up meat, and that he would run for the nearest steak if I weren't looking. Of course, I *am* the one who inspired David to become vegan, but he read the same books I did and reached the same conclusions. I'm grateful my becoming vegan didn't create tension in our relationship, but for many women it does, and that has a lot to do with socially assigned gender roles whereby women still tend to do the grocery shopping and cooking and feel obliged to feed their *hungry man* all manner of meats. Personally, I've heard from more vegan women whose husbands have followed them into plant-based eating than those who have not, but I've also heard from plenty of women for whom the tastes and preferences of their family take precedence over their own—compelling them to prepare meat for their husbands, male partners, and sons even if it disgusts them.

I certainly don't begrudge anyone for wanting to please their loved ones or for choosing the path of least resistance. I get it. We've all been pressured to conform to the status quo at one time or another. It *is* easier to go with the flow, blend in, eat like everyone else, and look like everyone else, but the question we have to ask ourselves is *At what cost?* At the cost of our own values? At the cost of our own health? Those are pretty high costs, in my opinion. That's not to say we have to rock the boat every chance we get, but what's the point of having opinions and values if we don't manifest them in our behavior or defend them when they're being undermined? We all want to make a difference. We all want to leave our mark on this world, do something meaningful, live a purposeful life, provide for our loved ones, protect the things we care about, contribute something important. Everyone says they want to make a difference, but

I think we forget that in order to *make a difference*, we may have to *do something different*. Only people who are willing to assert their individuality and act on their personal beliefs will actually have an impact.

One of our major tasks as we mature from adolescents to adults is to navigate the difficult waters of differentiating our personal identity and values from those we internalized from our parents and the broader dominant culture. This is what it means to grow; this is what it means to be human—negotiating the tensions that inevitably arise in our social circles when we emphasize one identity over another and reconciling all the contradictions that come with being multifaceted humans. Walt Whitman wasn't the only one who contained multitudes. We all do. In other words, if being vegan didn't threaten our belongingness to a particular group, something else likely would.

> In order to make a *difference*, we may have to do something *different*.

Identity is never fixed; it's variable, flexible, and reflexive, and it continues to develop throughout the course of our lives, shaped collectively by all of the groupings that give rise to who we are. We're continually shifting the placement and priority of our many identities—as men, women, mothers, fathers, husbands, wives, daughters, sons, Christians, Jews, Muslims, atheists, progressives, conservatives, Italians, Americans, Cubans, African Americans, humans—and vegans. We don't have to exclude one for any other. We can absolutely live harmoniously within our existing communities while adhering to our many personal values and multiple identities. We can—and should—embrace being a Puerto Rican Catholic Male Vegan or a Gay Black Vegan Atheist or whatever various identities we claim. Just as we don't have to abandon our vegan identity in favor of the others, we also don't have to abandon our other identities in favor of being vegan. Guiding our friends and family to see that eschewing animal flesh and fluids is not antithetical to our existing group memberships, but rather part and parcel of it, will help them better understand our new behaviors and thus not see our veganism as a rejection of them.

## THE DARK SIDE OF TRIBALISM

Although we may feel excluded for being vegan because it doesn't jibe with the accepted norms of a particular group we belong to, we may want to examine where *we* create divisions between ourselves and those groups as well. Do we overemphasize our vegan identity to the exclusion of others? Do we respond to rejection with rejection? Do we avoid community gatherings where meat and animal products are served? Even if we do these things in the name of self-preservation, our friends, family members, or other peers may still feel judged or rejected themselves because of them. As much as we dislike when people make generalizations and assumptions about vegans, we may be unaware that we're making generalizations and assumptions about those who aren't. Do we talk about people in dichotomous terms—as being either *vegan* or *not vegan*, as if no other identities exist or matter? Do we foster an us-versus-them, good-versus-bad, vegan-versus-nonvegan mentality? Indeed, the identity-forming process is as much about drawing distinctions as it is about highlighting similarities, but when differences are exaggerated, it can move us further and further away from our once-beloved, once-safe communities, leading to strained relationships and severed bonds.

As we've seen, belonging to a group of people with common beliefs and values is a fundamental human instinct, and tribalism—having a strong feeling of identity with and loyalty to one's group—can play out in positive ways, such as when we align with a particular sports team, religion, sorority, fraternity, country, gender, race, military branch, profession, political party, pro- or anti-movement, or any other special interest group. Tribal affiliation can provide communal strength and foster trust, cooperation, and even love. But tribalism—like all human instincts—can have a dark side. Tribalism becomes problematic when we see our group as superior to—rather than just different from—another group. Or when we dwell on what divides us from another tribe rather than on what unites us within our own. Tribalism's negative aspects are in play when we make being vegan look like a club or a clique that's exclusive to those who think and act exactly like we do, or when we perceive anyone who isn't vegan as the enemy. For some "ethical vegans," their vegan identity supplants even their *human* identity, such as when they denounce billions of their fellow humans by idealizing the extinction of the human race. (*After all,* they would say, *it's humans who are wreaking all the havoc on animals.*) The ugly side of tribalism can keep potential vegans away and push existing vegans out.

> Tribalism is problematic when we make being vegan look like a club or a clique that's exclusive to those who think and act exactly like we do.

To remain a vegan, then—and a joyful vegan at that—means cultivating relationships in *all* of our communities: in both our smaller tribes of family and friends and in our larger tribes of culture and kind. As we discussed in Stage Three, some relationships change and some fall away, but not all do, and some that are strained can be rebuilt. I'm not suggesting we stay in relationships that are toxic, shaming, abusive, or unsatisfying, but we need to nurture our place in the other communities to which we belong. We may be vegan, but we remain coworkers, neighbors, friends, daughters, sons, uncles, aunts, parents, grandparents, siblings, and fellow humans.

## FINDING YOUR LIKE-MINDED COMMUNITY

Once we've established what we need in order to feel confident being vegan within our existing communities, it's natural and necessary for us to want to find, build, or join a community of people who share our vegan values. One of the reasons vegans yearn for connection and community is to find a respite from the cruelty they see all around them. Just knowing you're not alone and that other people think and feel as you do—that there is a commonality of experience—is often enough to feel connected. Finding a like-minded community might entail simply following other vegans on social media, reading blogs, or listening to podcasts. I've personally heard from thousands of people over the years who told me that when they first became vegan and found my podcast, videos, and books, they considered me a friend who made them feel connected and less isolated.

"I know it's a bit silly, since I've never actually met her, but I feel like Colleen is my friend. I live in an area of rural England where I'm pretty isolated in my veganism, but because of Colleen's work and her support and wisdom, I don't feel alone."

"Listening to your podcast has been so helpful in keeping me from feeling like I'm lost or alone—or losing my mind!! I'd be listening and sometimes just burst into tears, shouting, 'Yes! That's exactly how I'm feeling!' Your podcast makes me laugh and cry and gives me the strength, patience, and focus I need to navigate as a joyful, kind, and compassionate vegan, especially when so many around me are not!"

"Becoming vegan has been the best decision I've ever made in my life. I feel truly liberated and truly connected with everyone around me—both human and nonhuman animals; however, the journey isn't without its very difficult moments. In the mere six months since I became vegan, I've gone through many emotional ups and downs, and I've often felt incredibly isolated. Thankfully, I found your work to keep me connected and less alone."

"I have yet to meet a vegan in real life, but hearing you read the love letters you've received from people all around the world, you showed me that I was not alone and that there was indeed hope for this world."

While hearing your voice echoed in someone else's and feeling that you belong to something bigger than yourself is essential, it is not necessarily *enough* to stay vegan—or at least to remain a joyful vegan. As grateful as I am that my work provides comfort and support to people all around the world, it's still just a bridge; I'm no substitute for a proper community. So while I encourage you to find and follow virtual role models, I recommend also that you join online and offline forums and groups filled with real people with whom you can identity, kvetch, and problem solve. Being part of a supportive community of people who share the same joys and heartaches, victories and challenges, pleasures and concerns is critical to staying vegan. Search online for local vegetarian/vegan/animal organizations, meetups, happy hours, groups, VegFests, or potlucks. Go to Meetup.com to see if there are any near you; start one of your own if there's not. As isolated as you feel, you may be surprised to find others in your town or county who feel exactly as you do and who are yearning to meet others like them. Many popular social media websites enable you to filter by location, so you may be able to turn some of the online relationships you're cultivating into real-world friendships. (This can also empower you as an advocate. Evidence suggests that when individuals realize they are not alone in their beliefs about an issue that may be considered contentious in the public eye, they become more willing to speak out.)

Whatever groups you find, you may want to watch from the sidelines for a bit to gauge the tone and content before you chime in. If you join one vegan (or plant-based or animal advocacy) group and find it doesn't match your perspective or personality, try another—or try several at once. It might take some time to find your tribe, but don't give up. And don't assume that just because you've found some that aren't to your liking that they're all the same. They're not. Also don't assume that a few cranky members are representative of the entire group. They're probably not.

Online groups can be a great resource for making vital and intimate connections, but I very much recommend joining those that have rules of engagement that explicitly emphasize respect and civility over those that don't. You may be relieved to find a community of vegans or animal advocates but dismayed to witness attacks, judgements, and vitriol within those communities. After all, some vegans are still stuck in the anger stage, some have turned their vegangelism into fundamentalism, and some wear their "vegan" badge as a way to signal their virtue to the rest of the world.

We may understand *why* some vegans act this way (read all the previous chapters), but the effects are not innocuous. It's a turnoff not only to potential vegans but to existing vegans as well. Perpetual bad behavior stokes divisions and could have the unintended consequences of pushing other vegans back into their meat-eating ways. I'm not saying that everyone who witnesses conflict in a vegan community returns to eating animal flesh and fluids or that recidivism is the fault of angry vegans, but if people feel less accepted by other vegans who profess to be kind and compassionate and more accepted by nonvegans who don't judge their every move, they will naturally gravitate toward the people who make them feel good. Baumeister and Leary didn't just find that the need to belong is *fundamental* to our human surviving and thriving; they found also that "satisfying the belongingness motive requires that two aspects of relationships be met: The first part is that people need to have positive and pleasant—not negative—interactions with others.

> Being part of a supportive community of people who share the same joys and heartaches, victories and challenges, pleasures and concerns is critical to staying vegan.

The second part specifies that these interactions cannot be random but, rather, should take place as part of stable, lasting relationships in which people care about each other's long-term health and well-being."[11]

In other words, belongingness isn't satisfied simply by virtue of affiliation; it's satisfied when we form and maintain positive, supportive relationships. It's not enough to be a vegan among vegans; we need to feel accepted and secure as well. This applies also to how we respond when someone announces they're no longer vegan. In Faunalytics' survey on recidivism, "more than a third (37 percent) of former vegetarians/vegans indicated that they're interested in resuming a vegetarian/vegan diet. Of these individuals, more than half (59 percent) said they are likely or very likely to do so."[12] That's a reason to be hopeful, but given vegans' reactions to ex-vegans on social media, I'm not sure the latter will feel there is a place for them if they want to return. My hope is that by gaining insight into why some vegans become ex-vegans, we can not only avoid the traps ourselves, but also be more sympathetic and understanding to those who do lapse—and be ready to welcome them back when and if the time comes.

> It's not enough to be a vegan among vegans; we need to feel accepted and secure as well.

## DISAGREEMENT MEANS DIVERSITY

That's not to say that even in a safe environment of compassionate vegans there can't be disagreement; of course there can—and should be—room for differences of opinion. Just because we share a common ethic of compassion and wellness doesn't mean we have to share the same viewpoints on other matters. Being inclusive means welcoming different opinions and perspectives. Unfortunately, the binary identity divisions currently dominating politics (us/them, in-group/out-group) are all too prevalent in the vegan community as well. You're either welfarist or abolitionist. You're either plant-based or vegan. You're either vegan for health or vegan for animals. If you're vegan for health, you can't call yourself "vegan" (according to the vegan police). If you're vegan for animals, you're probably a "junk food vegan" (according to whole food, plant-based eaters who avoid processed foods).

We profess diversity, but what we really seem to prize is homogeneity—particularly homogeneity of thought and ideology. There is a presumption among some vegans that if you're vegan, you're also liberal, socialist, atheist, feminist, intersectionalist, progressive, and leftist—and that if you're not these things, you're unwelcome, or at least you don't really belong. I've heard from a number of vegan men and women who feel there is no place for them in the vegan community because they don't fit into the above categories.

If believing that it's better to eat plants rather than animals is the only thing we agree on, that's enough. That's a lot. That's really what *vegan* means. Some vegans, however, have made it their mission to change the definition of what it means to be vegan, asserting that to be truly vegan, it's not enough to just forswear animal flesh, fluids, and fabrics. According to them, you also have to tick these boxes:

1. Be an animal activist.
2. Identify as liberal, feminist, intersectionalist, anticapitalist, atheist/agnostic, etc.
3. Renounce foods that are not also fair trade, palm oil–free, organic, and GMO-free.

Though the intentions are good—inspiring more people to get involved to help stop violence against animals as well as creating connections between animal abuse and other social issues—the unfortunate result is a narrowing rather than a broadening of the vegan pool. As you add criteria to the definition of veganism, fewer and fewer people qualify. And by making the door through which people can walk even smaller, fewer and fewer people will cross the threshold—or even want to. The number of people who meet the basic and widely understood definition of veganism is already small enough. Do we really want to make it smaller?

Being respectful and welcoming of different political, social, or ethical views doesn't make us hypocrites; it makes us diverse. Inviting diversity means also inviting (and accepting) diversity of ideas, perspectives, lifestyle choices, and life experiences. There are plenty of organizations, associations, and groups you can join that celebrate conformity of thought, and that's fine; there's a place for them online and in our real lives. But many vegans aren't necessarily looking to be advocates or activists; they're just looking for a community where they don't feel like a freak for not eating meat, dairy, and eggs. That should be the only price of admission.

To those who argue that we shouldn't welcome or accept people who—though they may not be *eating* animals—may be contributing to harm in other ways (wearing leather, buying personal care products that were tested on animals, going to the zoo, etc.), I say this: we're all on a journey. The process of awakening is just that—a *process*. I've heard from thousands of people who stop eating meat, dairy, and eggs for health reasons; then, at some later point, their hearts and minds become open enough to start considering rejecting other forms of culturally accepted animal abuse (which I address more in Stage Eight—Stretching Your Comfort Zones). It may take time, but it's *their* journey—not yours—and a sure-fire way to impede their progress is to call them "fake vegans" and judge them for not "getting it" more quickly.

The same applies to those in the "plant-based" community who criticize overweight vegans and excoriate anyone who eats oil, sugar, gluten, or processed foods. Not only is it unkind, it's also not your business. Everyone's journey is their own. You can certainly model positive eating habits and provide inspiration and information, but I encourage you to temper any desire to criticize and judge. People don't respond positively to either, and they certainly don't respond well to body-shaming. The bottom line is that the desire to not hurt animals and to live healthfully is universal, and those who espouse them should be embraced regardless of weight, color, creed, country, class, culture, or political affiliation.

Being—and staying—a joyful vegan means having a broad notion of what it means to be . . . any of the things we are. None of our identities—cultural, religious, gender, human, etc.—are static. Being a joyful vegan means giving ourselves permission to embrace *all* of our identities, even as they morph and change and expand. It means spending energy not only noting differences but also recognizing similarities and acknowledging that the individuals in our respective identity groups are complex beings, not one-dimensional stereotypes. Being a joyful vegan means being confident in our vegan identity without undermining our other identities; it means embracing a broader definition of diversity to include diversity of thought and ideology. It means fostering relationships in all of our communities and valuing all of our identities. There is no prescribed profile of what a vegan looks like, dresses like, worships like, votes like, or acts like. Or at least there shouldn't be. We all contain multitudes.

> Being welcoming of diversity means also welcoming diversity of ideas, perspectives, and life experiences.

*Stage Seven*

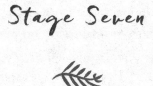

# Finding Your Voice

## *How to Talk to a Hunter*
## *(Or Anyone Else with Whom You Disagree)*

Knowing others is intelligence; knowing yourself is true wisdom.
Mastering others is strength; mastering yourself is true power.
—Lao Tzu (trans. Stephen Mitchell)

B efore Farm Sanctuary's northern California sanctuary closed and all the animals were relocated to their new homes, I used to spend a great deal of time there—volunteering, documenting the animals' stories, and just lovin' on all the furred and feathered residents. During one particular stay, I volunteered for a very difficult task that would

189

become a touchstone for measuring my own communication skills. Abutting one side of Farm Sanctuary's property is government-owned land on which a "dove shoot" takes place each year. Hardly worthy of being called a *hunt*, this event consists of shooting birds either out of the sky as they fly to and from their roosting sites or while they perch in trees. Needing to stay in good stead with the local ranching community and dedicated first and foremost to the safety of their own animals, Farm Sanctuary had no recourse to stop the annual shoot from taking place, but it *could* post people to "patrol" the fence to make sure no birds were shot once they flew on their side of the property line and to potentially help any injured birds who fell on their land. I volunteered for the patrol.

I braced myself for what promised to be two very challenging days where I would be watching live doves being shot out of the sky, one after another. I wasn't there to protest. I wasn't there to obstruct. I was there to play a very specific role on behalf of Farm Sanctuary and on behalf of animals. And I was scared to death—scared of what I would see, of what I would feel, of how I would react, and of how I would perceive the men who would be killing these birds. I could feel my heart pounding, my pulse racing, and my stomach churning as a group of men dressed in camouflage arrived just before sunrise, bringing guns, coolers, folding chairs, and dogs into the large open field housing the few tall shrubs where the birds roosted.

I assessed my options. I knew that from my side of the fence, I could very easily communicate with my body what I couldn't say with my voice; I could stand with my arms folded, my body tense, my face frozen in a scowl. I could watch these men with justified anger and righteous indignation, stoking my ire and cultivating my disgust. Feeling powerless to stop the slaughter, I figured I could at least let them know with nonverbal cues exactly what I thought of them. As the sun rose and the men took their positions in the field, I made a decision to do just the opposite. I decided to exhibit with all of my body and all of my mind the compassion that was lacking in the field that day. I decided to stand in a completely open posture—with my arms at my sides or behind my back—literally and figuratively exposing my heart. I decided to keep my face soft and my stance light, and I created a mantra that I repeated in my head over and over and over during the course of the day: *May compassion fill your hearts, my heart, and this field. May compassion fill your hearts, my heart, and this field. May compassion fill your hearts, my heart, and this field.* It was challenging, to say the least. Every time I heard a gunshot or listened to the men laugh and cheer when a bird fell to the ground, I kept repeating: *May compassion fill your hearts, my heart, and this field.* As tears filled my eyes, I said it again and again—sometimes speeding up the cadence of my words as if the momentum of the repetition would increase the efficacy of it.

The way the dozen men were situated in this large field, I couldn't see all of them, and only a few could see me in detail, but I'm certain they could see my open stance as I stood and strolled along the fence line. They were also aware that I didn't shout at them or react, even when some of them made antagonizing comments. I didn't respond, I repeated my silent incantation, and I tried to remain open. At one point my friend, who at the time ran the sanctuary, drove up to bring me food and tea. One of the guys shouted from across the field, "Hey—I'd like to order some hot coffee! Can you get us some breakfast?" I shouted back: "All you have to do is say you'll go home, and I'll make you a delicious, hot breakfast—with coffee." They laughed and said, "Touché." And we all carried on from sunset to sundown: me, struggling to maintain my compassion; them, killing birds.

But as the day wore went on, I could feel something shift—subtly but noticeably. As the sun moved, so did the men, and at one point, the shooter who had been across the field from me had moved over to the fence line exactly next to where I stood. It was unnerving to be so close to what I perceived as the antithesis of everything I believed in, to see the human face of someone whose actions were anathema to me. He sat on his cooler eating a sandwich, as I stood just a couple of yards away. I purposefully didn't retreat. I squatted down to pet his dog through the opening in the wire fence and asked the man the dog's name. He told me, and we had a brief exchange about something I don't remember. I stood up and stayed close by, all the while trying to fill my heart with as much compassion as I could muster. Then he turned to me and said, "This must seem awfully crazy to you." I quietly responded, "I don't understand. I just don't understand." And we both fell silent.

As the sun began to set and the men started to pack up their things, he turned to me again and said goodbye. I responded in kind and wished him well, and he walked away—not haughtily, just quietly. I was stunned, and my heart was bursting. I had vowed to fill the space we had shared that day with the compassion that I perceived was lacking, and in return my heart was filled with the same. It was palpable. The next morning, I went out again and kept the same stance, which was even more difficult because this time they had brought children with them, a young boy and a young girl. I didn't stay long this time—I was needed elsewhere—so another volunteer took my place. I was relieved I didn't have to see more birds get shot, but in a strange way I was disappointed to lose the chance to plant more seeds of compassion in that field. I tried to do so in my mind with each distant gunshot I heard.

Later, the volunteer who had taken my place told me that a couple of the guys had asked why I wasn't out there that second day and indicated that they had been moved by my presence the day before. When they were leaving, one of the guys asked her to convey his best to me—all of which confused her very much since she had no idea what had happened the day before. She said that they were genuine in their well-wishes and that the whole exchange was very strange; she said she felt no hostility from them at all. If anything, she said, it was almost as if they were embarrassed by their reason for being in that field. My friend, who had witnessed many dove shoots over the previous decade she had been managing the sanctuary, said they shot many fewer birds that weekend than she had ever seen. Perhaps there were fewer birds to shoot; I don't know. I certainly don't take any credit for that. Nor do I believe I had a profound impact on any of these men.

What I am certain of is that I was the model of compassion that I wanted to be—that I profess to be, that I encourage others to be. I verbally and nonverbally manifested kindness, nonviolence, and nonjudgment, and they were returned to me in kind—merely by virtue of my *embodying* compassion, if not by my compassion's recipients. In expressing, exhibiting, and exuding compassion, I experienced compassion. If I had expressed, exhibited, and exuded anger, outrage, and judgment, I would have experienced anger, outrage, and judgment. Not only would that not have felt very good, it wouldn't have changed a thing. My sadness during the dove shoot was apparent; I didn't have to shout at the shooters to make that clear. I knew there was nothing I could do to stop those doves from being killed or to make those men go home, but what *was* in my power was how I chose to comport myself and how I chose to communicate. And that brings us to the next stage in our journey: communication and the quest to find your voice.

## HONING YOUR VOICE

Developing communication skills is necessary for every area of our lives, but as vegans and advocates it's especially important because veganism, animal consumption, and animal exploitation are all sensitive issues in our society, often making people—vegans and nonvegans alike—defensive, emotional, irrational, and fearful. Whether online or in person, whether from strangers or friends, hostile comments, insensitive jokes, passive-aggressiveness, and myths and misconceptions all come with the territory, and learning *how*, *when*, and *if* to respond to them is one of the key components of effective communication. Every vegan or vegetarian has been on the receiving end of someone who's trying to catch you— someone who's trying to find fault with your choices, or a hole in your logic. You're asked to defend your reason for not eating animals, you're asked the same questions over and over, and you're expected to answer dispassionately, but with grace and poise.

As we've seen, this is the case even if you don't consider yourself an advocate. As soon as you say "I'm vegan," you open yourself up to curiosity, questions, and challenges; it's one of the reasons some people purposefully avoid saying they're vegan. They don't want to call attention to themselves; they don't want to have to answer for what they feel are private decisions; they don't want to be attacked or criticized. I address strategies for being effective *advocates* in the chapter on finding your place (Stage Nine), but my hope is that my suggestions for effective *communication* may inspire even the most reticent of vegans to find their voice. As I demonstrated in my story above, communication is not simply about what we say, or even our body language. It starts with what we think. And that is my first suggestion for effective communication:

## 1. Create intention.

Communication starts long before we even open our mouths. How we perceive a person, a situation, or ourselves has an impact on how we engage. My decision to see the dove shooters as vessels into which I could pour my compassion rather than as enemies or adversaries shifted my perception of them, my behavior, and thus our interaction. This approach can be applied to any and every situation we're in and to every person we encounter. Simply calibrating our thoughts toward one intention over another will affect the outcome. For instance, I hear from many vegans who ask me how they should order food when they're with nonvegans at a nonvegan restaurant. "I don't want to appear difficult or problematic, so how can I ask for what I want without making a scene or calling attention to myself?" It all starts with our perception. If we perceive ourselves as being problematic or difficult, then that comes across in our language and demeanor. Holding that perspective, we apologize profusely (for simply asking for what we want). If we *think* we're high-maintenance, that's what we'll project. Whereas if we're confident that it's perfectly reasonable to ask a few questions about a menu item, then that's what we'll project and that's usually what will be received. That doesn't mean someone still won't think you're difficult or high-maintenance, but it won't be because of your actions. It will be because of their own perception, and you don't have any control over that.

Creating intention is especially important when it comes to talking about being vegan, which some people automatically interpret as proselytizing—and indeed, as we've seen, some vegans do set out to proselytize. I can't control how someone interprets what I say, but I can make sure I'm clear and honest about the intentions behind what I say. Even as a vegan advocate, my intention is not to *make people vegan*. It's not in my power to *make* anyone do anything. All I can do is speak the truth and trust that it will inspire others to act on their own values. Whenever I set out to do my work—whether I'm writing an article, working on a book, speaking to a group, or talking to someone one on one—in my mind, I make sure I'm clear about my intention, and my intention is this: to raise awareness about violence against animals, to be their voice, and to speak my truth.

> My intention is not to *make people vegan*. It's not in my power to *make* anyone do anything. All I can do is speak the truth and trust that it will inspire others to act on their own values.

That's it. I believe intention is everything, and people individually and collectively are smart enough to see right through you if you appear false to them—if you appear to have a hidden agenda, or if you seem to be saying one thing but really mean another. Having a clear intention about your goal and making that goal about *truth* rather than *outcome* will make you a successful, effective communicator 100 percent of the time. It's the difference between approaching someone and thinking, "What can I say that might make them vegan?" and approaching someone and thinking, "What can I say that will reflect the truth?"

Whenever I'm about to talk to someone—whether in a public lecture, an interview, or a private conversation—I have a little mantra I say in my head, and it goes like this:

> *Put the words in my mouth, the love in my heart, and*
> *help me tell the truth with integrity and compassion*
> *and without attachment or expectation.*

Creating an *intention mantra* of your own will help you let go of expectations about how others will react and what they will do with the information you share. None of that is yours. Maybe your intention is to be open, nonjudgmental, patient, and sincere. Calibrating that in your mind first—especially before a potentially difficult or emotional encounter—will make all the difference in terms of how you interact, how you engage, and how you are received.

## 2. Practice active listening.

Because vegans are expected to be experts in all things related to food, nutrition, history, animal husbandry, etc. to justify our choices, we often feel pressured to *say* the right thing—the thing that will inspire someone to stop eating animals. Not only does that set us up for disappointment, it also means we're focused more on talking than on listening, which is an oft-neglected aspect of communication. Active listening entails fully concentrating on what is being said rather than thinking about what you're going to say in response. Hearing is one thing. Listening is another.

My model for active listening came about after my husband, David, and I attended our first Japanese tea ceremony here in northern California. The experience is about so much more than just drinking tea; it's about being fully present in the moment, in the space. As a guest, you're invited and encouraged to appreciate and comment on every element that has been chosen especially for the occasion—the tea utensils, the flowers, the hanging scroll (and its calligraphy and calligrapher), the food, the kimono, the teapot, the tea bowls, the tea scoop, the tea. When the tea is served, the host kneels directly in front of you and bows. You bow back. You bow to the person to your right and thank them for letting you go next. You bow to the person to your left and ask to be excused for going before them. You take a sip of tea. You acknowledge the sensation, the color, the flavor. Every gesture is full of intention and presence and awareness and respect. This has become my model for communication: it's what David and I call *facing forward*—being fully engaged, remaining fully present, giving your undivided attention.

One of the ways active listening can be beneficial, especially when we encounter what may seem like absurd or illogical questions, is as a way to understand what's really being asked underneath what appears on the surface. Even though people sometimes do play the "gotcha" game, I think in general people are really curious about veganism and just don't know what to say, so they wind up asking what may sound like a silly question to you but is, on a deeper level, a genuine question to them. For instance, when someone asks a vegan, "Why don't you care about plants? They have feelings, too," It's unlikely that they're actually concerned about any potential emotional trauma experienced by cauliflower or carrots. I think what they're really asking is "How crazy is this vegan thing? How far does it go? Where do you draw the line? If I try to do something right, what about all the things I will do wrong?" If I respond by saying that being vegan is about doing the best we can despite living in an imperfect world, answering their question on that deeper level, they may be more inclined to consider my viewpoint. If I respond by quoting scientific studies to try to dispute their claim about plant feelings, I've lost. I've lost them, because that wasn't what they were really asking, and I've lost my own foundation, because now the discussion has moved away from talking about what we *do* know: that animals unquestionably feel pain and undoubtedly suffer due to our anthropocentric practices and philosophies. Actively listening means being better able to keep the conversation on course.

A cornerstone of engaged listening is getting clarification before responding. Too often in conversation, we react to something that's not even being said, which is why so many arguments wind up with someone declaring, "That's not what I meant!" We often hear what we want to hear, what we expect to hear, and what we're piecing together in our own mind. One way to avoid this is to confirm with the person you're talking to: "What I hear you saying is X. Is that correct?" Give them the opportunity to either confirm or clarify, then ask again: "Before I reply, I just want to make sure I understand you correctly. What I'm hearing you say is X. Is that right?" The goal is to get to the point where they say, "Yes, that's what I'm saying," so you can then proceed with your response. This sounds like a lot of time before you can even reply, but I would argue that your time is better spent on clarifying up front than on arguing about things that were never even said in the first place.

## 3. Understand the power of nonverbal language.

Obvious though this is, it bears emphasizing: effective communication is not about verbal language alone; it comprises body language as well. The profound experience I had during the dove shoot was a direct result of the nonverbal cues I projected rather than about anything I said.

Our outward body language reveals our inner thoughts and affects both how we communicate those thoughts and how those thoughts are received. Here are some things to consider:

- Be aware of your body language. You may not even realize habits you've formed that you may want to modify. Start with awareness of how you stand, if you fiddle, what your face says while you're listening. For instance, do you cross your arms in front of you? Doing this doesn't always send a negative message or mean we're not listening, but sometimes it can. The same goes

for crossing our legs. Pay attention to your own body language
to determine what signals you might be giving off.

♦   Make eye contact. Unconsciously, we tend to avert our eyes while
we're talking to someone, but our eyes do indeed reveal quite a
lot about who we are and what we're thinking. We can read each
other much better when we look straight into someone's eyes,
which is why face-to-face communication will always trump
online communication. Social media, email, text messages, and
other online forms of communication certainly have their place
in our relationships, but for meaningful conversations or difficult confrontations, in-person is always the way to go.

♦   Don't interrupt, and avoid finishing other people's sentences.

## 4. Check your verbal intonation.

Another argument for in-person communication has to do with the fact
that tone, inflection, and cadence of speech—all important elements of
communication—are completely absent in email, texts, and online conversations. If you can't hear the tone in someone's voice, it's very difficult
to gauge the spirit of what they say, and it is too easy to overreact to what
may be an innocent or inoffensive comment. Emojis can provide visual
markers of our emotions that text alone cannot achieve, but they're not
always enough. So when communicating, make sure your tone is consistent with what you're saying. If there's a chance your tone was misunderstood, pick up the phone or go see the person. Going back and forth via
email or tweets to clear up a misunderstanding does not often lead to a
productive dialogue and can even make things worse.

## 5. Ask questions.

Not only does asking questions make others feel important and heard,
it also helps you understand exactly what is being said. Vegans often feel

they have to have all the answers—and perfectly articulated answers at that. Of course being able to respond with facts, science, and interesting information is part of communicating (and debunking myths), but it is neither possible nor reasonable to know everything about all the disciplines veganism touches. Asking questions like "Can you tell me more about that?" or "Can you elaborate on that further?" are ways to explore and clarify ideas, and it makes people accountable for what they say. This is especially helpful if someone is perpetuating a myth or if they declare they could never go vegan. Asking "What are you afraid would happen if you did go vegan?" or "Have you ever considered trying something like a 30-Day Vegan Challenge?" may be more effective than arguing that they *could* go vegan if they really cared. If someone tells you they hunt, you could ask them, "When did you first start killing animals? What did it feel like? How does it feel now?" Or if someone says, "I could never give up steak, but I gave up pork because I heard pigs are like dogs," you might ask about their dog and help them identify the traits they value in their dog, then point out that cattle have the same traits. Or if someone spews pseudoscience about meat consumption, instead of trying to argue about a study you haven't looked at yourself, you can say, "I haven't heard about that. Can you tell me more about it?" Or even, "I don't think that's true, but where did you hear that?" or "I can't really believe that's the case, can you?"

## 6. Have a sense of humor.

Laugh. Lighten up. Relax. Yes, even when someone makes a stupid vegan joke. Because violence against animals is a very serious issue, talking about it can make people uncomfortable. One of the ways humans deal with discomfort is to deflect it by making a joke. A joke might seem insensitive, but often it actually comes from a place of sensitivity. Sometimes people make jokes because they don't know how else to respond. Or they're uncomfortable. Or, yes, because they want to goad you. In any case, it really helps to laugh. Levity can lighten up the most tense situations. It demonstrates that you can stand up for what you believe in and still have a sense of humor. You can be serious about a serious cause without taking yourself so seriously all the time. Your laughter doesn't undermine animal suffering (or your commitment to end it); in fact, the animals you want to help are better served by your joyful existence more than they are by miserable martyrdom. After all, people are more attracted to joy than they are to misery.

> You can be serious about a serious cause without taking yourself so seriously all the time. People are more attracted to joy than they are to misery.

## 7. Speak your truth, then step back.

Detachment (or *nonattachment*) is considered a virtue in many Eastern religions as well as in the Western philosophy of the Stoics, and it is a guiding principle in my work as an advocate and as a human. The two-thousand-year-old *Tao Te Ching* is regarded as the cornerstone of the Taoist tradition, and short though the book is, it could be whittled down further to just two words: *let go*. Almost every one of the eighty-eight short chapters cautions against *clinging, expecting, grasping*, even *hoping*—regarding attachment as the source of all discomfort, and detachment as the source of serenity.

"Express yourself completely, then keep quiet."

"Just do your job, then let go."

"Stop trying to control."

"Do your work, then step back."

"He [who is in harmony] lets all things come and go effortlessly, without desire. He never expects results; thus he is never disappointed."

"Things arise and she lets them come;
things disappear and she lets them go.
She has but doesn't possess,
acts but doesn't expect.
When her work is done, she forgets it.
That is why it lasts forever."[1]

The three principal leaders of ancient Stoic thought—Seneca, Epictetus, and Marcus Aurelius—all had similar things to say in their own writings, stressing Stoicism's central concept: that human beings cannot control life, only their responses to it. Expectation, in the form of fear as well as hope, will lead to disappointment.

From Seneca (c. 4 BC–65 AD):

"True happiness is to enjoy the present, without anxious dependence upon the future, not to amuse ourselves with either hopes or fears but to rest satisfied with what we have, which is sufficient, for he that is so wants nothing."

From Epictetus (c. 55–135 AD):

"We cannot choose our external circumstances, but we can always choose how we respond to them."

And from Marcus Aurelius (121–180 AD):

"You have power over your mind—not outside events. Realize this, and you will find strength."

"If you are distressed by anything external, the pain is not due to the thing itself, but to your estimate of it; and this you have the power to revoke at any moment."

"Receive without pride, let go without attachment."

This concept is difficult to comprehend and even more so to implement, especially for those who perceive *letting go* as weakness and for activists who see it as passivity. Nothing could be farther from the truth. Being clear and standing firm in what you say but remaining unattached to how someone *reacts* to what you say is incredibly empowering and liberating.

To be clear, speaking your truth and stepping back doesn't mean throwing a Molotov cocktail into a conversation, then saying, "Hey, whatever you do with that isn't my problem. I'm not responsible for how you react." Being unattached to outcome doesn't give us license to be demanding or rude or ungracious, and it doesn't authorize us to stop someone else from speaking their truth. It means that we speak up without being *attached* to how our words affect another person—whether for better or for worse. As a result, we feel lighter, more resilient, and more serene.

## 8. Disagreement is not disrespect.

I grew up surrounded by people who interpreted disagreement as disrespect; who inferred that if you argued with them, you were making a judgment about their intelligence; who took everything so personally that they perceived your expression of your beliefs as an attack on theirs. These are not strategies for effective communication, and yet we do this all the time in our in-person and online interactions with one another. We've become so accustomed to the dichotomous paradigm of "I'm right/you're wrong" that we have abandoned the possibility that we can simply disagree and still remain in the same room. Politely and confidently saying "I disagree" is a skill worth learning.

1. "We're on the same page on X issue, but I don't agree with you on Y."
2. "It seems we have different points of view."
3. "I've drawn different conclusions."

4. "I've made different observations."

5. "While I still think we have different approaches/perspectives/beliefs, I understand yours a little better now. Thanks for sharing it with me."

F. Scott Fitzgerald famously said, "The test of a first-rate intelligence is the ability to hold two opposed ideas in mind at the same time and still retain the ability to function." In other words, humans are complex creatures with *many* viewpoints as well as *changing* viewpoints. We can celebrate one aspect of a person while disagreeing with another. Hunters, for instance, are easy targets for vegans and animal advocates, some of whom lump them all in a box called "evil," but can you imagine saying to a friend whose father, brother, or uncle hunts: "Hunters are evil. How can you even still talk to your father/brother/uncle?" My friend would most likely say, "My father/brother/uncle is not evil. He's actually a good person with a big heart. I don't know how he's able to hunt, and I have a really hard time with that aspect of what he does, but he's a good father/brother/uncle. I wish he didn't do that one thing, because it isn't congruent with the rest of who he is, but I still love him." The bottom line is we can see and appreciate the whole of a person while disagreeing with and even despising an aspect of what they believe or how they behave. Creating a space to hear someone else's

> Creating a space to hear someone else's beliefs, especially ones you don't share yourself, doesn't mean your beliefs will be diminished.

beliefs, especially ones you don't share yourself, doesn't mean your beliefs will be diminished. If anything, they will be strengthened. You may even learn something.

Even when we agree to disagree with someone so a conversation doesn't turn into World War III, that doesn't mean we have to be so self-effacing as to not stand up for what we know to be true or right.

We've all been in scenarios when someone shares misinformation we might not have the exact rebuttal for, and that makes us feel that we "lost" the argument or "lost" the upper hand. But it feels that way only if we look at every conversation as a battle. If we're committed to planting seeds rather than winning an argument, then I believe that honesty, confidence, and humility are some of the best ways to do this.

You might concede, "I haven't read that particular article/I can't speak to one person's experience not thriving on a plant-based diet, but I do know that you'd be hard-pressed to find a doctor who tells their patients to cut back on the number of vegetables they're eating and to increase their consumption of animal products, and the research bears this out." You might not have read that particular blog post or article or whatever it is they're citing, but you can still remain confident about the overall issue. "I can't relate to the points you said were made in that article. I've never had those experiences, and I've never felt better. Perhaps the person who had health issues wasn't making the most nutrient-dense food choices." Anecdotes and a single documentary film are not substitutes for science.

## 9. Speak from the "I."

Someone once asked me why I speak in terms of "we" or "I" even when referring to things I don't partake in anymore. For instance, I might say "When we buy animal products, we're supporting a violent system." Obviously, *I'm* not buying animal products, but the reason I speak from the "I" is because I want people to relate to me, and I don't want them to feel dictated to. Not only is it true that I, too, once ate animal products, it's also true that people don't respond well to being told they're doing something harmful. As we discussed in chapter one, we choose willful blindness in order to preserve a perception of ourselves as being good and kind, and I would be directly challenging that perception if I said, "When *you* buy animal products, *you* are supporting a violent system." Although that might be true, the question is *Will it be heard?* Not likely. People tend to get defensive when they feel they are being criticized, chastised, or told what to do. Maya Angelou said it best: "People will forget what you said and did, but they will never forget how you made them feel."

Note the difference between "Don't you know that animals are being tortured? Why don't you care that animals raised for your food are being subjected to pain and suffering?" and "When I ate meat and other animal products, I had no idea animals were being tortured. I was able to convince myself that animals being raised for my food weren't being subjected to immense pain and suffering." I've received countless emails from people who see a huge difference in responses to their social media posts when they make this slight but significant tweak. When you speak from the "I," information is conveyed in a way that makes it relatable rather than as a personal attack. It makes difficult information more palatable.

## 10. Speak to people as individuals.

Vegans don't like when generalizations are made about them, and yet they make generalizations about nonvegans all the time. When speaking to someone, try to see them as an individual—not as someone who eats a certain way, votes a certain way, or works in a particular industry. In other words, don't use a one-size-fits-all approach when talking to people. Adapt your content to the person or people in front of you—even if they ask a question you've heard a million times. In a way, you are actually hearing it for the first time, because it's the first time you're hearing it from that particular person in that particular moment, and it may indeed be the first time they've asked someone that question. By seeing each encounter with each individual person you meet as a new and exciting opportunity, you will have a more authentic and satisfying experience.

I might add one more suggestion: *practice*. Aristotle famously said, "We are what we repeatedly do. Excellence, then, is not an act, but a habit." Being a great communicator means practicing being a great communicator. It is a skill like any other. The only way to get good at it is to do it often, learn from and rectify your mistakes, and implement in future conversations what worked well in past ones.

The bottom line is we can speak up for animals without speaking down to humans. We can stand up for something we believe in without standing over others. Communicating effectively means finding our voice and expressing ourselves, our desires, our needs, our wants, and our values in a way that is productive, effective, truthful, and compassionate; and it means knowing the difference between using words that provoke thought and words that provide shock. The former shifts paradigms; the latter exists for its own sake. The way we communicate either draws people in or pushes them away. The better we are at communication, the stronger and more diverse our community will be—one that consists of fellow vegans, aspiring vegans, and supportive nonvegans.

> We can speak up for animals without speaking down to humans. We can stand up for something we believe in without standing over others.

## Words Matter

### *Vegan, vegetarian, or plant-based?*

Need more evidence that how we say something makes a difference in how people respond? A study by the World Resources Institute's Better Buying Lab found that the public was more likely to embrace vegetarian/vegan meat products when the products were labeled "meat-free" instead of "vegetarian" or "vegan," and many companies are indeed adopting "plant-based" as an alternative to "vegan" and "vegetarian" on their packaging and in their marketing materials.[2] As a result, they're seeing increased sales among meat-eaters. According to the Good Food Institute, "Researchers at the London School of Economics found that when vegetarian items were moved from the menu's vegetarian section and listed on the main section, sales went up by more than double (56 percent)."[3] Similarly, according to a recent survey summarized in a report called "Consumer Trends in the Food and Beverage Industry," "the word 'vegan' reduces foods' appeal for more consumers than other common labels like 'diet,' 'sugar-free,' or 'gluten-free'."[4]

Why do "meat-free" and "plant-based" seem to go over better than "vegetarian" or "vegan" with the general public? First of all, "plant-based" focuses on what a product *includes* rather than what it *lacks*, but more than that, industry experts think "plant-based" just doesn't carry the same negative baggage that the terms "vegetarian" and "vegan" do. Some people may have had negative experiences with vegetarians and vegans. Others, perhaps due to social norms, guilt, or other reasons, may simply look down on all things "vegetarian" or "vegan." Especially for people older than thirty, the term might conjure up memories of a flavorless tofu burger they tried back in college rather than today's more vibrant vegan offerings.

Second, the public may see vegetarians and vegans as a distinct group of people quite different from the average American—and themselves. The labels "vegetarian" and "vegan" tend to say more about who someone is than just about what they eat. "Plant-based," on the other hand, reflects a food preference rather than a moral position. A poll of 1,163 social media users suggested that "plant-based" is perceived in a more positive light than "vegan." The former is seen as more of a proactive dietary choice characterized by flavor, health, and flexibility; the latter is seen as a lifestyle choice characterized by deprivation, rules, and allegiance to a cause.[5]

I don't think this means we should never use such terms or stop calling ourselves "vegan"—many of these studies and surveys relate to food labels and not people—but it's helpful data to have. Know your audience and how they react to certain words.

*Stage Eight*

# Stretching Your Comfort Zones
## *Expansion of Awareness and Skills*

What can take place without change? What then is more pleasing
or more suitable to the universal nature? And can you take a
hot bath unless the wood for the fire undergoes a change? And
can you be nourished unless the food undergoes a change?
And can anything else that is useful be accomplished without
change? Do you not see then that for yourself also to change is
just the same, and equally necessary for the universal nature?
—Marcus Aurelius, *Meditations*

There's no denying that becoming vegan requires a massive shift in perception and a change in behavior that most humans resist. Change is one of the most difficult things for humans to cope with—even when that change is positive—and most of us are unaware of how habit- and routine-oriented we are until we actually try to change our patterns. As a species, we naturally value comfort and predictability and find solace in the familiar, and our habits provide this—they make us feel safe and secure. They allow us to tackle everyday challenges and keep our stress levels in check by giving us structure we can rely on and rules we can adhere to. From an evolutionary perspective, habits save us time and free up our mental energy so we can focus on more complex thoughts and goals. In these ways, our habits are a blessing. They can be a curse, however, when the support they once provided becomes a crutch, a limitation, and a barrier to anything new. In these ways, our comfort zones become a prison; routines become rote; habits become addictions.

Clinging firmly to old patterns, people, and perspectives, we are terrified to let go—to change—until we're absolutely forced to, and indeed it's often only some kind of trauma, tragedy, or unexpected event that knocks us out of the familiar: a death, a job loss, a breakup, an illness. Some of us experience our vegan awakening despite never having sought it out, stumbling into it because of an accident, a doctor's recommendation, or a physical ailment. Some of us go into it not just reluctantly, but kicking and screaming. We anticipate restriction, expecting to have very few options when it comes to food especially, but once we make the leap, we discover the most exciting and unexpected aspect of becoming vegan: that it naturally expands your awareness and your skills.

What you think will be a restrictive way to live and eat actually turns out to be more expansive than anything you could have imagined—in terms of the perspectives you discover, the options you have, and the actions you can take. You see yourself and the rest of the world through a much broader lens and inevitably ask, *Why didn't I do this sooner?*

Exploring unfamiliar territory becomes a quest, and what you thought would be a challenge becomes an adventure.

You try cooking for the very first time (and realize you like it!). You buy your first food processor or high-powered blender and experiment with new ingredients. You try new cuisines and create new recipes. You become more interested in nutrition, take a certification course, or start a vegetable garden. You begin to challenge your body in new ways—by taking up running or bodybuilding, yoga or Pilates.

> The most exciting and unexpected aspect of becoming vegan is that it naturally expands your awareness and your skills.

It's not just your behavior that changes; it's your thinking, too. You discover new interests, you challenge old ideas and notions, and you feel your relationships with others deepen. You recognize the connections between this issue and other social issues and begin to learn about the history of the vegan and animal protection movements. If you became vegan for health reasons, you start to see animals in a new light. If you became vegan for ethical reasons, you begin to want to eat more healthfully. Although one door has closed, many more have opened; everything feels new and novel, especially when it comes to food and eating.

I've heard people say they don't want to be vegan because they would get bored eating the same foods again and again, as if monotony is unique to vegans. Everyone—regardless of whether or not they eat meat, dairy, and eggs—gets into food ruts. Most of us buy the same foods week in and week out, go to the same restaurants, order the same favorite dishes, and rarely venture out of our comfort zones. In fact, research shows that because we cluster in tight, like-minded communities and increasingly receive advertising messages customized specifically to our preferences and past purchases, our tastes are narrower than ever—even though we have more options than ever.[1] There's nothing wrong with having a familiar routine and rotating favorite foods—as long as that rotation includes a variety of healthful vegetables, grains, fruits, nuts, and seeds to ensure you're taking in the greatest number of nutrients—but we *all* need to make a habit of injecting flavor, fun, and diversity into our routines, no matter how we eat. And that just requires *being open*, which is one of the gifts of becoming vegan and one of the secrets to staying vegan.

One of the things that tend to happen very naturally when you become vegan is that your palate and preferences expand and an entire world of food opens up—foods that were available to you before you became vegan but that you ignored because you were already set in your ways. When you shift your gaze from one direction to another (from animal products to plants), you realize there are cuisines, flavors, textures, aromas, and experiences you never tried before. You discover Ethiopian, Burmese, Indian, and Thai cuisines. You're more culinarily adventurous and try making new dishes at home. You realize there's a vegan version of everything, including artisanal cheeses and meatless meatballs, hot dogs, and burgers—even seafood.

"I used to cook *zilch* before becoming vegan. I never really learned and did not enjoy it at all. Since going vegan, I've discovered so many new ingredients. It's changed my whole lifestyle and even made me like cooking!"

"Another benefit to this new change is that I learned how to cook!!!"

"Once we moved into our apartment, I immediately ordered my first vegan cookbook and began ascertaining what foods would be replacing the eggs and cheese we so heavily relied on. Within weeks, I was so thrilled with how many new foods I was discovering! Not that I didn't know what they were; I just wasn't accustomed to eating many of them—like tempeh, tofu, seitan, parsnips, and Swiss chard."

"Thank you for making what I thought was going to be a miserable experience into a joyful and empowering way of life. The food I have been preparing has been colorful, nutritious, varied, and delicious. I've never been a confident baker, but your book has changed even that! I couldn't be more thrilled—and neither could my coworkers, who get to eat the treats I bring to work!"

"I love cooking and have found new pleasure in discovering new foods to eat and new ingredients to play with."

"I've learned so much on my journey so far. I feel empowered and full of energy, and better yet, a whole new array of flavors has opened for me."

"What I'm loving about this vegan journey is that I'm eating food and seeing recipes that are global in nature. I'm learning more about other world religions and cultures that have different dietary preferences that align with the values of eating vegan. I feel my heart is becoming more open and connected to people of other countries like I've never felt before."

I often put "vegan food" in quotation marks to make the point that "vegan food" is food we already eat and love—it's fruits, vegetables, nuts, seeds, beans, lentils, mushrooms, herbs, and spices. Yet because of their association with vegetarians and vegans, some of these foods tend to be compartmentalized as foods *only* vegans eat, especially tofu, seitan, and tempeh—as attested in some of the letters above. These foods have been enjoyed in their countries of origin—China, Japan, and Indonesia, respectively—for hundreds and thousands of years by vegetarians and nonvegetarians alike, but in the West, we don't tend to eat them until and unless we become vegetarian or vegan. Another food you don't tend to eat until you take the vegan plunge is cheesy-tasting nutritional yeast—aka "nooch" or "gold flakes," as it's been affectionately nicknamed—a nonlive yeast fermented on molasses. I had never heard of it before becoming vegan, and now I don't eat popcorn without it. But truth be told, in the family, culture, and time I was raised in, I had also never heard of dates, quinoa, or sushi. It wasn't until I became vegan—and thus began trying new foods and cuisines—that such delicious foods became a regular part of my repertoire. That's not to say I would never have tried them had I not become vegan, but once meat, dairy, and eggs were no longer options, it encouraged me to explore other gastronomic realms.

"Vegan food" is food we already eat and love—it's fruits, vegetables, nuts, seeds, beans, lentils, mushrooms, herbs, and spices.

As your palate expands, foods you never thought you'd try become favorites, and foods you never knew existed become staples. In fact, a lot of things you never thought you'd do become part of your routine and things you'd never thought you'd buy become countertop favorites:

- You buy a pressure cooker and swear it's changed your life.
- You make your own plant milks.
- You buy a soy milk maker and try your hand at making tofu.
- You make "nice cream" ("ice cream" made simply from frozen bananas).
- You buy a slow cooker and an air fryer.
- You make kale chips and "sweet potato toast."
- You make desserts with avocado and black beans.
- You eat hemp seeds, chia seeds, spirulina, and spelt.
- Quinoa becomes your go-to grain.
- You drink kombucha (a fermented tea beverage).
- You discover aquafaba (the liquid in a can of chickpeas, used in place of eggs in baking).
- You photograph and share every meal you eat.

Again, none of these things are unique to vegans, but there's no denying that once you venture into this world, you embrace new and novel things.

It's not just tangible experiences like eating and cooking that are expanded; having removed a veil from in front of their eyes, many vegans talk about seeing things more clearly and feeling things more acutely. As many of the following letters reflect, when you become vegan, you tend to feel an increased connectedness not only to your own values but also with other humans, other animals, and other causes, as you recognize the links between violence against animals and violence against humans. You endeavor to reduce waste, use less plastic, and live more mindfully. Your relationships deepen, your empathy expands, and you feel more attuned to the natural world—and more inclined to protect it.

"The world looks so different to me—the awareness I now have is astounding. I'm finally living my truth, and I cannot tell you how different I feel inside and out. I have an astounding appreciation for all life on this planet and for each and every creature. I have never been happier with a choice that I have made, and I will never, ever look back."

"I feel in alignment with my values. I'm learning to stand up for myself and my beliefs in a way that I would never have expected. I'm learning that it is okay to ask for what you want (nicely, of course!) and to have strong opinions. I'm finding my voice not just in connection with veganism, but in so many areas of my life. I don't feel deprived; a world of choice and love has opened up around me."

"Being vegan changes your life; you literally observe everything around you with a different perspective—through a different set of eyes. Your awareness increases, and it's like being able to see for the first time."

"I started out thinking this was going to be a healthy diet change, and I now truly see how very important this is for our world. I now see the connection to climate change and to the health of our planet. I am even more committed than when I started and more passionate about it than I ever thought I would be."

"I feel like my heart opened more to my fellow humans, and I have to say this empathy developed tenfold *after* I became vegan."

"Learning about the oppression animals experience makes you aware of all of the humans who are also oppressed. I truly found my humanity when I went vegetarian—and more so when I became vegan!"

As we settle into our newfound veganism, our reasons for staying vegan also expand. If you *become vegan* for ethical reasons, you invariably learn more about eating, cooking, and nutrition; if you *become vegan* for health reasons, your heart and mind open to learn about the ethics. The fact is, there are a number of doors through which people can walk to *become vegan*, and not all of them appeal to everyone, but once you're *in* and looking through a new lens, you begin to make connections you weren't able to make before. Willful blindness is a powerful thing; it requires us to be very self-protective and avoid seeing the forest for the trees. But once you stop participating in the behaviors that create the cognitive dissonance (that is, once you stop eating meat, dairy, and eggs), you're able to let down your guard and become more vulnerable, more open, and more aware. What you may have avoided looking at before becomes just one more reason to support your decision. Most vegans will say that though there may have been one thing that sparked their desire to be vegan, they remain so for many reasons. And indeed, we don't have to pick just one—we can care about many things at the same time.

"For me, the ethical component was the most important one, so I guess I would have become vegan no matter what, but thanks to your helpful advice, I also started to think about health, nutrition, and how fun it can be cooking delicious food at home!"

"Unlike other people who have written to you, I have not been a life-long animal lover. I don't have pets now and frankly in the past didn't really like other people's indoor pets. I didn't become vegan because of my affection for animals; I became vegan because of my belief in justice. However, what's amazing now is I can't pass a dog walking down the street with his human companion without stopping to admire or pet him or her. This has opened up a whole new appreciation for non-human animals that is as surprising to me as it is to everyone who knows me."

"I was initially motivated to change because of the shocking environmental impact of the animal agriculture industry which I had been largely ignorant of . . . then I became increasingly affected by the disgraceful treatment of animals (which I probably knew about but, like everyone else, chose to bury my head because I don't like change). Now I feel proud to be part of a community that boycotts this horrific slaughter and astounded that it doesn't even feel like a sacrifice. I'm loving the challenge of experimenting with new ways of cooking and feeling excited about the obvious health benefits that vegan living affords. It's win-win, and I still have so much more to learn!"

"I didn't truly believe in the 'compassion' element of changing my diet until I completed the 30-Day Vegan Challenge. I considered myself a healthy eater before the challenge and had previously cut all meat but fish out of my diet. It was more difficult to do that than to go vegan because I didn't have any ethical ties to vegetarianism. But what happened was so surprising and enlightening: once I started taking care of my health, I was able to see the need for me to take care of our environment and all living creatures."

You may have become vegan for *one* reason, but you *stay* vegan for many, and in fact, research indicates that having more than one reason may actually increase the chances that you'll remain vegan. According to Faunalytics,

> People who maintain a veg*n [vegan or vegetarian] diet are more likely to have multiple reasons for doing so than those who lapse. In our recent study, current vegetarians and vegans reported a broader range of motivations for their diet than did lapsed veg*ns. While a majority of former veg*ns cited only health as their motivation, a majority of current veg*ns identified a number of motivations: health, animal protection, concern for the environment, feelings of disgust about meat/animal products, and taste preferences.[2]

Although I do believe that people's perspectives expand naturally once they stop eating meat, dairy, and eggs, I have noticed that people who are motivated by health can sometimes be reluctant to learn more about the ethical issues related to animal agriculture—perhaps because they feel they don't need any other motivation since they've already made a huge change, or perhaps because they don't want to witness animal cruelty (who does?). Some purposefully identify as "plant-based" rather than "vegan" to avoid being seen as sanctimonious or moralizing, as reflected in this excerpt from a letter I received: "When people found out I was vegan and would roll their eyes, I would quickly say, 'Oh, I'm not that kind of vegan. I'm just doing it for my health.'"

Not everyone stops eating animal products for the same reason, and that's fine, but just keep in mind that if you intentionally limit your reasons for not eating meat, dairy, and eggs, you may increase the chances that you'll start eating meat, dairy, and eggs again. You don't have to identify as "vegan" if you don't want to, but there does seem to be value in at least having more than one motivation for eschewing animal products, and that may require being willing to look at how the production of meat, dairy, and eggs affects the animals themselves.

A recent study that focused on "lifestyle choices of individuals following a vegan diet for health and ethical reasons" found that people who go vegan for ethical reasons are more likely to remain vegan than people who go vegan for health reasons.[3] According to the authors of the study, "Ethical vegans reported following the diet for an average of about eight years, whereas health vegans kept to the diet for about five and a half years." While the exact reasons are unclear, the findings reminded me of a story I heard many years ago on National Public Radio about how empathy or, even more specifically, *awareness that someone else suffers because of your actions* is the most motivating factor when it comes to behavior change.

The study focused on which factors contributed to success when it came to quitting something like nicotine—and staying quit. The people who had the most success remaining smoke-free were the ones who had internalized exactly *how* their smoking hurt those they loved. The study looked at people who hadn't had a cigarette for many years but who started desiring one not from a physical need—after all, the nicotine was well out of their bodies—but from an emotional need. Despite the temptation to smoke, what stopped them from picking up a cigarette again wasn't concern about their own health but rather the awareness that if something happened to them because of their smoking (lung cancer, heart attack, emphysema), it would cause immense pain and suffering to their family members. One woman said she was overwhelmed with sadness when she thought of how devastating it would be for her daughter to lose her. That was enough to keep her from lighting another cigarette.

Something similar may be happening for people who become vegan for ethical reasons: they may be more motivated to stay vegan because of their awareness that returning to a nonvegan lifestyle would cause suffering to another. Of course, it's not that people who become vegan for health reasons are selfish (a common insult hurled at "plant-based dieters"); it may be simply that they have not yet borne witness to the suffering of animals. Being open to looking and learning about how animals suffer on factory farms and in slaughterhouses may be beneficial in preventing a return to eating meat, dairy, and eggs.

To be fair, it's not that there is *no* recidivism among people who become vegan for the animals. There are plenty of reasons why both groups return to eating meat, dairy, and eggs, but this one might be a clue to reducing recidivism among "health food vegans." It's also one of the reasons I recommend periodically bearing witness to the plights of animals. Not only does it serve as a reminder of what may have inspired you to become vegan in the first place, it can also serve as additional motivation for *staying* vegan—whatever your original reasons were.

# Finding Your Place

## *Advocacy and Activism*

"I wish it need not have happened in my time," said Frodo.
"So do I," said Gandalf, "and so do all who live to see such
times. But that is not for them to decide. All we have to
decide is what to do with the time that is given us."
—J.R.R. Tolkien, *The Fellowship of the Ring*

Having stretched our comfort zones, honed some new skills, and expanded our awareness, the next questions we tend to ask are *How can I help? How can I use my skills and knowledge to be part of the solution? Where do I fit into this whole thing? What is the best use of my time? What is the best use of my money?* Sometimes the answers lead us to a new vocation, sometimes to an avocation. We may become activists, or we may use our income to support activists—or both. But this stage in our journey isn't simply about figuring out what to do for a living or what type of advocacy to engage in. It's about finding our place in the context of this larger cause—whether our motivation is health, animals, or the environment. To be clear, you don't have to become an advocate to remain vegan, but chances are you'll be inclined to align your commitment to veganism/plant-based eating with other aspects of your life.

Finding your place doesn't necessarily mean you have to quit your job, change careers, work for a vegan organization, or take to the streets with placards and petitions. Finding your place might mean working at a job totally unrelated to veganism at which you're happy, successful, and well paid but that enables you to financially support people who have chosen to do this work full-time. Even if you don't consider yourself an activist in the formal sense of the word, you *are* making a difference by virtue of not contributing to the inherently unsustainable, inhumane, unhealthy practices of the animal exploitation industries, and whether you intend to be or not, you are an ambassador of compassion and wellness.

Still, if you feel that being vegan is not enough and you want to delve into more active advocacy, there are many ways to get involved. As you begin to explore your options, I encourage you to keep in mind that the question isn't necessarily "What is the best type of advocacy to get involved in?" It may be "What type of advocacy is the best for *me*?" As you venture down this path, here are a few things to consider:

1.  Answering the question "What type of advocacy is the best for me?" means thinking about what you're good at, what you love, and what excites you most. You're going to be most effective if you're coming from a truthful, authentic, joyful place.

2.  There may not be *one single* answer for you; there may be several things you're interested in. If so, I think you'll find a common thread running through them. Perhaps your answers are all related to communication, education, technology, or legislation.

In other words, if you have several interests, it might be helpful to identify the *category* they all fit into to help give you a bigger picture of where you want to devote your efforts.

3.  Whatever your answer is to the question "What type of advocacy is the best for me?" be open to the fact that it may change. You may change your mind, get burned out, or just get bored, but that doesn't mean you have to throw out the baby with the bathwater. If you're doing one type of advocacy and you're finding it taxing, emotionally draining, or less gratifying than it used to be, the best thing to do is try something else rather than stop advocating altogether. You might discover a new talent or passion, or you may find something you're even better at. It's okay to try one type and then another.

Always be open to evaluating and reevaluating what you're engaged in to make sure it's satisfying and effective—not draining and depleting. Often, we think we have to keep doing something because we've already invested time and resources, or we're afraid to switch to something else because our identity has become defined by a particular type of activism. When it comes to effective advocacy, we need to continually ask:

→  Is this working?
→  Is this effective?
→  Am I happy?
→  Am I burning out?
→  Are there changes I can make within this type of activism to make it better, more sustainable, more effective? If not, do I need to try something else?

Nothing is ever so good that it's above a little revision. Effective advocacy means being flexible, open, curious, and self-reflective. We will never have all the answers, but we should always be asking questions.

The work I'm doing today is similar to the type of advocacy I was drawn to early on in terms of the larger categories—writing, communication, information, outreach, education—but the forms have changed and the mediums continue to evolve. My very early advocacy involved volunteering at a county animal shelter, where I socialized cats and cleaned their cages. I started out going one day a week, then two, then several, because it was heartbreaking to think that if I didn't show up, nobody was going to interact with the cats or give them some time to stretch their legs outside of their cages. (Guilt certainly drives a lot of advocacy, which is why we need to make sure we pause for self-care.) I had become vegetarian around that time, and in an effort to raise awareness about the different forms of socially sanctioned animal abuse I had come to care about, I began making little brochures and flyers about various issues: puppy mills, vivisection (using animals as research tools), and vegetarianism. This was before the internet, so I typed out the names and telephone numbers of various organizations on each brochure and distributed my handmade materials to passersby at the mall—before I was stopped for doing so because I didn't have a permit. I had no idea what I was doing, and I didn't know any other activists; I just needed to do *something* to speak up for animals.

Several years later, after moving to California and becoming vegan, I stepped up my activism. Every weekend, I would head out for the streets of Berkeley, set up my TV/VCR, play a loop of *Meet Your Meat*, and hand out copies of *Why Vegan?* pamphlets. I had countless conversations with compassionate consumers who wanted to stop participating in these atrocities but whose minds were filled with myths and misconceptions about veganism. I realized they understood *why* becoming vegan was optimal, but they didn't know *how* to make the transition. So, I started teaching vegan cooking classes in my city of Oakland. I had no formal culinary training, but I knew enough to help those who knew less than I did. In addition, I organized events with speakers (such as my hero, John Robbins), hosted film screenings of documentaries, led youth groups in discussions about veganism and on tours of animal sanctuaries, and began giving talks at schools and churches, while also continuing to teach vegan courses and cooking classes that were open to the public every month. I taught these classes for ten years.

Because I wanted to reach more people than those who attended the cooking classes, I raised the money to produce a cooking DVD to sell and distribute.* Once that was in motion, I started writing, producing, recording, and hosting a podcast—in 2006, long before most people, including myself, really knew what a podcast was. Although it was my dream to be a published author, I never thought my first book would be a cookbook, but since my goal was to give people the tools and resources they needed to become and stay vegan, I felt it was a necessary labor of love. Same with the second book and the third. After writing cookbooks, I turned to writing books to help people transition to being vegan and to live with conviction and compassion—including the book you're holding in your hands. I also started writing opinion pieces for various publications and radio shows, and I became (and remain) a regular contributor to my local National Public Radio station. I began doing regular TV segments and speaking to audiences all around the world—at VegFests, conferences, and universities—and I created The 30-Day Vegan Challenge online program to give people a multimedia experience as they made their transition. My political engagement also increased as I began working with local officials to pass animal-friendly legislation, and I cofounded a political action committee to help elect animal-friendly candidates. I've also come full circle and once again volunteer with an animal rescue organization, socializing cats.

When I left graduate school in 1996, I wasn't even vegan—I was barely vegetarian (more like pescatarian)—but I already knew I wanted to dedicate my life to animals. I vividly remember saying to my fellow

---

* Shout-out to animal advocate extraordinaire Alka Chandna, who I initially taught the classes with and who generously helped me produce and host the cooking DVD.

graduating classmates, "I don't know what it's going to look like, and I don't quite know what *form* it's going to take, but my goal is to do something related to writing, teaching, advocating for animals, and helping people at the same time." Those threads continue to run through my work today. I knew what I was fairly good at, and I knew what I was passionate about, but I didn't know exactly what the work was going to be. I think it's fair to say that when I graduated with a master's in English literature, I didn't envision myself teaching cooking classes, creating recipes, or screening slaughter videos on the streets of Berkeley. Even though I could have worked for an animal or vegan organization, I always knew I wanted to work for myself, so I set out to do just that. As I was advocating in all the ways described above, I also worked full-time as a content director for a nonprofit organization unrelated to animal issues; it was a good job doing good work, but my heart wasn't in it, and after a few years, I left to turn my avocation into a vocation.

I was able to do this because I never stopped asking, *What am I good at? What do I love? What is there a need for? What is effective? How can I use my skills, gifts, and interests to be the most useful?* I encourage you to ask yourself these types of questions whether you want to find your place as a volunteer or as a professional. Here are some questions to get you started; add them to your own journal or word processing software and take some time to work out your answers.

- → What moves me?
- → What do I love?
- → What am I good at?
- → What are my gifts?
- → What are my skills?
- → What are my talents?
- → What gets me excited?
- → What am I passionate about?
- → What do I see as a gap that only *I* could fill?

If you love writing, *write*. Write a blog, a book, magazine articles, opinion pieces, letters to the editor, or even legislation.

If you love talking to people, *talk*. Speak at high schools and universities, start a podcast, make videos.

If you love cooking, *cook*. Create recipes, write a cookbook, teach classes, start a business, open a cafe (but be sure to partner with someone who has business skills if that's not your forte).

If you're an artist, *create*. Draw, paint, illustrate, sculpt, design.

If you're a musician, *make music*.

If you're a filmmaker, *make films*.

If you love politics, get involved, support animal-friendly candidates and legislation, run for office.

Everyone has a contribution to make, whether as an independent contributor or as a volunteer for an individual influencer or a larger organization.

It is worth saying, however, that effective long-term advocacy is not just a matter of figuring out what you love and what makes you feel good. It's also about figuring out what you *don't* love and what *doesn't* make you feel good. Some people are perfectly comfortable attending protests or demonstrations. Some people hate writing; some are scared to death of public speaking. Don't do something you loathe just because you think you should. That's not to say we should never stretch our comfort zones and try something different, but if you try something and still feel intimidated, inadequate, or uncomfortable, there's probably a better place for you, and by stepping away you open up a space for someone else who is better suited. You also free yourself up to find where you belong.

As for choosing specific types of activism, I mention some below, but you can also search online for ideas; reach out to organizations and influencers to see what their needs are; read books like Mark Hawthorne's *Striking at the Roots: A Practical Guide to Animal Activism*, Stephanie Feldstein's *The Animal Lover's Guide to Changing the World,* and Jennifer Skiff's *Rescuing Ladybugs: Inspirational Encounters with Animals That Changed the World* for inspiration. And keep in mind that you don't have to found, work for, or volunteer at a nonprofit organization to find your place or have an impact. The recipient of your precious time (and money) might also be an independent content creator, a podcaster, a blogger, or a grass-roots activist. The primary difference between a nonprofit organization and a sole proprietor is simply that the former doesn't have to pay taxes. Tax-exempt status doesn't make someone better organized; it just means they have to comply with a few rules, so keep an open mind when it comes to figuring out who you want to donate to, work with, or volunteer for.

# A VOCATION

If you *do* want to work on behalf of veganism or animals full-time as a solo entrepreneur but you are in a job you can't currently quit, you can begin to build your second vocation as you work in your first. It may mean working two jobs while you create the business you want; it may mean finding an investor or a business partner; it may mean taking out a business loan—it all depends on the type of work you want to do. You may want to get certified, take a course, or earn a degree. Figure out what you need to do, make a plan, and put one foot in front of the other. Fear is what stops most of us from making a change: fear of not having enough money, fear of not succeeding, fear of succeeding, fear of the unknown. If any of that sounds familiar to you, I encourage you to take the time to write down what your goals are. Having a more concrete vision of your future can make it feel less intimidating.

- → How do I envision myself spending my days?
- → Do I see myself working from home or in an office?
- → What kind of contribution do I see myself making?
- → What types of jobs am I best suited for?
- → What blocks do I need to clear to make the first step possible? The second step? The third?
- → What am I afraid of?
- → What am I excited about?

Get clear about what you want and what you want to do. This exercise is not only useful for those who want to work for themselves; it will provide clarity even if you want to work for someone else. Once you have a better understanding of what you want to contribute, you will find that there are plenty of different positions at many different vegan companies, vegan organizations, and animal protection organizations you can apply for.

## EARNING A LIVING

Another important question often gets neglected by those whose motivations are altruistic:

→ How much money do I need to make to live comfortably without having to worry about paying my bills?

I hear from so many large-hearted people who are working in a job or on a project that promotes veganism or animal protection (or who are eager to do so) but who feel they need to say, "I'm not doing it for the money. I'm doing it for the animals" (as if anyone goes into animal advocacy for the cash). They emphasize that they're working for free or running on so shoestring a budget that they can't make ends meet or pay anyone to help them, because they want to devote everything they have to the larger cause. Poverty and self-sacrifice become emblems of magnanimity: the less you make, the more it shows you care—a sentiment even some vegans use to criticize fellow vegans or animal protectionists who make salaries greater than they think they deserve. There's a notion that if you generate money from noble work, you're probably *really* a greedy mercenary, and if you *do* want to do good work in the world, you ought to renounce the desire to live comfortably. I don't think these ideas are unique to vegans and animal advocates; I think they abound in other movements as well, especially in those inclined toward anticonsumerism, anticapitalism, and socialism.

To say we humans have a schizophrenic relationship with money is an understatement. When we don't have it, it's all we think about. When we do have it, we want more of it. When we have more, it's never enough. When others have it, we're envious; when others don't have it, we blame those who have it for keeping it from those who don't. The bottom line is you can both do good work in this world and want financial security at the same time. You don't have to choose one over the other. That's not to say we can't make sacrifices for the larger cause, but asceticism need not be a prerequisite for advocacy. Don't be ashamed for wanting to make money. Neither the animals nor the humans who benefit by our work need us to be monks as much as they need us to be strategic. They don't need us to be poor as much as they need us to be successful, visionary, and effective—with enough money to enable us to do our work without the distraction of worrying about having enough money.

> Asceticism need not be a prerequisite for advocacy.

## START WHERE YOU'RE AT

News flash! You don't have to change careers to use your voice for animals; there are countless ways to advocate in the framework of your current job, whether you're a software consultant, a trucker, a teacher, a real estate agent, or a restaurant worker. Whatever you do—as either your vocation or avocation—you have an opportunity to make a difference:

→ If you're an interior designer, you can talk to your clients, colleagues, or company about wool, cashmere, and leather. If you work for someone else, you can request your company stop using these products in the name of environmental integrity and sustainability; if you're self-employed, you can make it your policy to work only with animal-free materials.

→ If you're employed by a corporation that provides food for staff events and meetings, you can influence the type of food that's served. Work with the Meatless Monday campaign (meatless monday.com) to implement it at your office.

→ If you're a nurse, doctor, or staff member in a hospital, perhaps you can screen movies like *Forks Over Knives* or encourage other staff members to take the 30-Day Vegan Challenge. Human resources may even provide incentives and benefits to those who take the challenge, especially if staff members can demonstrate improvement in their blood pressure, cholesterol, triglycerides, etc. after having made dietary changes.

→ If you're an attorney, you can donate some of your time to an animal law case. Contact the Animal Legal Defense Fund for opportunities.

→ If you're a hairdresser or work in a salon, you can transition to vegan, cruelty-free products.

→ If you work for a rodent expulsion service, you can switch to using only humane, catch-and-release traps.

→ If you're a filmmaker, you can try to make sure all the meals served on set are plant-based and refrain from using live animals or animal products during the shoot.

In fact, leveraging the power we have among the groups we're already affiliated with is the best way to effect large-scale change, whether we're talking about the local government officials we vote for, the companies we work for, the neighborhoods we live in, or the churches we are members of. Individuals are more willing to take risks and make changes when they're aligned with the status quo. Don't underestimate the influence you have to reset norms and therefore inspire new behaviors among the people and organizations you already have relationships with.

Certainly some jobs can be more challenging for vegans than others, especially those related to food; if you work in the food industry as a server, line cook, chef, baker, caterer, manager, or cafeteria worker, you're most likely handling meat, dairy, and eggs on a daily basis. If you're in this scenario and feel miserable doing your job, you have a few options:

1. Quit your job.
2. Quit being vegan.
3. Figure out a way to use the position you're in to advocate for veganism and animals.

**Option 1** would be self-destructive unless you have another job lined up. (Perhaps you can find a similar job in a veg*n restaurant.) As difficult as it may be to remain in a food-related job that requires you to serve or cook meat/dairy/eggs, animals aren't helped if you have no income, cannot pay your bills, and rack up debt. Make sure you have a plan before giving notice.

**Option 2** would be self-defeatist and illogical. It doesn't make sense to start eating meat, dairy, and eggs again just so you can stop feeling bad about handling meat, dairy, and eggs in your profession.

**Option 3** requires a bit of willful blindness, but it will enable you to do your work without losing your mind. When you're able and willing to leave your job, you'll do so, but in the meantime, there are a number of ways you can influence the restaurant you work at and the customers you serve. The most obvious way is to increase the plant-based offerings. Work with the management, owners, and/or chefs to get more plant-based options on the menu, arguing from the perspective of sustainability and profit and providing them with a number of resources to demonstrate the success of restaurants that have added more vegan options to their menus.

→ Organize a test taste with managers and staff that features products such as the Impossible Burger, the Beyond Burger, Just Egg, and Just Mayo—all brands that work with restaurants and commercial businesses. Contact the companies themselves for samples and to help find out what distributor your restaurant (or whatever type of food service company you work for) can order them from.

→ Reach out to Forward Food, which works with food service directors, chefs, and dietitians at universities, hospitals, major corporations, and restaurant chains, to add plant-based foods to their repertoire. Connect with them directly or check out their website (forwardfood.org) for recipes, resources (such as the Professional's Guide to Meat-Free Meals), and toolkits for university foodservice professionals, healthcare foodservice professionals, and restaurants. They also do culinary training.

→ Consult the Good Food Institute's database of food-service products at goodfoodscorecard.org; it includes photos, detailed information, and sales contacts.

→ There are countless stories of restaurant owners who become vegan and slowly start veganizing their establishments. You can do this, too! Check out Veganizer (theveganizers.com), a fantastic resource that includes a step-by-step guide for restaurateurs who want to fully or partially veganize their establishment.

Getting restaurants to add vegan options to their menu isn't enough, however. As we saw in the sidebar on page 207, research reveals that *how* items are marketed to customers makes all the difference in terms of how well they sell—or not.[1] Keep in mind that even if you don't work *for* a restaurant, you can still work *with* restaurants to help them implement these ideas. Restaurant outreach is a much-needed form of advocacy that anyone can do—wherever you live. Here are some suggestions you can encourage restaurants to implement to increase the sales of their plant-based options. (Some of these suggestions may also be useful to food activists, bloggers, recipe creators, and cookbook authors.)

→ Do *not* create a separate vegan menu. Rather, incorporate vegan items within the nonvegan items of the regular menu.

→   The name of the dish matters. Label menu items with words related to taste and enjoyment. Customers are more likely to choose "Zesty Chile-and-Citrus-Roasted Asparagus" over "Asparagus" and "Tangy Ginger Broccoli and Smoky Shiitake Mushrooms" over "Broccoli and Mushrooms."

→   Don't label the item as vegetarian or vegan. For example, title a plant-based burger "Impossible Burger" or "Beyond Burger" rather than "Vegan Burger" or "Veggie Burger." If it's not a commercial patty, call it something exciting like "Smoky Grilled Grain Burger" or "Mexican Bean Chipotle Burger." Only indicate that the item is plant-based in the description: "made with delectable plant-based ingredients for the discerning meat-eater."

→   As much as people profess to want to eat healthfully, they are less inclined to order something if it's labeled "healthy," "low-fat," "no-oil," or "low-calorie," as we equate these descriptors with "no flavor" and "no satisfaction." Instead, use descriptors like "indulgent," "decadent," "sinful," "rich," and "luxurious."

→   Increase the artistry of the dish's presentation. Studies show that *how* food is plated actually enhances the flavor—and thus increases the sales—of the menu item.

→   Aside from vegan burgers and nuggets, don't rely too heavily on seitan or tofu. They tend to have negative associations for nonvegans.

→   If you do add a commercial product to your offerings, contact the manufacturer so they can add your restaurant to the product finder page on their website.

Once the vegan items are on the menu and being marketed in a positive way, restaurants can further increase orders of their vegetarian or vegan options by using an effective little psychological trick. Social psychologists have known for a long time that when something is already being done by the majority of people, the rest of us think it must be a good thing, so we want to do it too. In other words, you can change a person's behavior by highlighting that other people changed *their* behavior. Social peer pressure for good! For instance, restaurants should advertise their new plant-based additions by saying something like "More and more people are trying our new burger." Restaurant servers should recommend the plant-based option and promote it as the special of the day, emphasizing its popularity: "Today's special—the Impossible Burger—is everyone's favorite." A recent experiment led by a Ph.D. student in psychology at Stanford University found that if a customer is told that other people are increasingly choosing the menu's meatless options, they are more likely to order a meatless meal.[2] The researchers worked with a burger restaurant near Stanford University to add to the menu a simple, unobtrusive message: "Our Meatless Burgers Are on the Rise." Affixed to the credit card machine was another: "We've noticed customers are starting to choose more meatless dishes." Over the course of seventeen days, these two small interventions resulted in an increase in the sales of meatless dishes of 1.7 percent, translating to over 180 people who chose the vegetarian option. When behaviors are presented as societal norms, it taps into our brain's deeply ingrained desire to conform to societal standards. If

> The word *advocate* comes from the Latin word *vocare*, which means "voice."

you're a server in a nonveg restaurant, just recommending the vegetarian and/or vegan options on the menu may work, but it might be even more effective if you did so by saying, "One of the most popular dishes is the [name of vegan menu item]" or "Our customers keep coming back for the [name of vegan menu item]," rather than simply "I recommend the [name of vegan menu item]." A subtle difference—but one that can have an impact.

Being a voice for animals at work—the word *advocate* comes from the Latin word *vocare*, which means "voice"—can be done quietly as well, even if it's just about protecting your own principles. When my husband was a software engineer, he was staffed on a project to build a website for a horseracing company. He told his manager that he didn't feel comfortable working on that project, and his boss happily put him on another. A friend of mine who works as a sound engineer at a radio station received a call from a journalist who wanted to rent the studio to interview a trophy hunter (someone who pays tens of thousands of dollars to kill large "game" animals). My friend works with many people whose values are not in alignment with his own, but he felt he just couldn't do this one in good conscience. He replied by saying that they were booked up and recommended a commercial production studio in the same city. Did that mean my husband's company didn't staff someone else on the horseracing project or that another studio didn't give studio time to a big-game hunter? No, but sometimes a little self-preservation is necessary as you're finding your vegan place in this nonvegan world. And remember, it's not just *who* you work for that provides you with an opportunity to advocate or not; it's *how* you spend your well-earned salary. With the money you make serving meat burgers, selling wool clothing, or recording interviews with hunters, you can support the vegan and animal protection organizations you care about. Consider it an offset.

Reconciling your veganism with the rest of your life is not always easy, and not everyone is an activist. It can be exhausting to see animal exploitation everywhere you turn and always feel obligated to combat it or guilty that you can't. As long as we're striving to live an ethical life, we will encounter difficult situations that test our patience and stamina. We're not always going to hit a home run in our efforts to advocate, but facing these situations can also make us stronger, wiser, and more resourceful. Will there be consequences when we speak out and step up? Yes. Will there

> Don't do nothing because you can't do everything. Do something. Anything.

be consequences when we don't? Absolutely. What's the alternative? Stop being vegan? Stop striving to live ethically? *Don't do nothing because you can't do everything. Do something. Anything.* We are not perfect people, and we do not live in a perfect world, but there is so much we can do in our individual lives to advocate for the things we care about. Even though we can't control the world, we can control ourselves. Choosing the type of advocacy that best suits us is one way to exert the power we have, but choosing what type of advocate we want to be may make the difference in how effective and how satisfied we will be.

## TEN HABITS OF HIGHLY EFFECTIVE ADVOCATES

Based on the success and mistakes of my own advocacy, as well as that of others I've observed and studied over the years, I've devised a list of characteristics of effective advocates. Putting into practice all or just some of these habits will not only help increase your efficacy, it will also help increase your happiness and peace of mind—especially if you're in this for the long game (which is one of the elements of effective advocacy: understanding that change takes time, perseverance, and patience). Some of these habits will come easily to you; some will need to be cultivated. Implement what you can, be open, and embrace the challenge.

### 1. Highly effective advocates manifest and model compassion.

We all know how easy it is to have compassion for those who agree with us, look like us, vote like us, and eat like us, but if we profess to be compassionate people, it means we have to strive to have compassion for everyone: the guilty and the nonguilty, the kind and the unkind, the good and the evil, the human and the nonhuman, the people we like and the people we don't, the vegan and the nonvegan. Authentic compassion means having compassion even for people who are not compassionate. Many people hear this and think that striving to have compassion for everyone—regardless of who they are and how they behave—means condoning inappropriate, dangerous, offensive, illegal, or violent behavior. They think it implies being a doormat, enabling abusive behavior, and keeping untrustworthy people in their life. None of this is what compassion is about. *Compassion doesn't condone bad behavior; it helps transcend it.*

> Compassion doesn't condone bad behavior; it helps transcend it.

Highly effective advocates recognize and truly believe that nonvegans are compassionate people, too. I've seen too many vegans (especially those who identify as "ethical vegans") write off nonvegans as cruel and insensitive, but I don't think that's the whole truth about people. I don't believe people wake up each morning trying to figure out how they can contribute to violence against animals that day. That doesn't mean there aren't sadists in the world doing horrific, unspeakable things, but the majority of people contributing to violence against animals are doing so out of ignorance and conditioning—not sadism and blatant cruelty. I think the truth is people are *so* sensitive that they don't want to believe that they're contributing to harm or violence against animals, and so they choose the easier route—ritualizing, rationalizing, and romanticizing their consumption of animals (see chapter one, "Don't Tell Me. I Don't Want to Know"). We humans have a great capacity to compartmentalize our emotions and support things we would never participate in directly—and then justify our behavior so we can sleep well at night. I know I did. But that doesn't mean the compassion isn't there. Before I became vegan, I was a compassionate person, but my compassion was blocked; it was conditional. Highly effective advocates know this and seek to guide people to their own compassion. But they also continually seek to be more compassionate themselves. The idea that only nonvegans compartmentalize their compassion is a false one.

We're *all* taught to compartmentalize our compassion and reserve it for only a select few, doling it out as one would limited, scarce rations—as if exercising it fully and authentically would deplete us of it or compel us to waste it on the "wrong people." And so we actually wind up *rationing our compassion*. We decide who is worthy of our compassion and who it should be withheld from, who deserves it and who it should be denied to. We see this play out in the ugliest of ways when animal advocates celebrate the death of hunters or prominent meat-promoting celebrities—cheering their demise in the name of *compassion* for animals. That's not compassion; that's vengeance. That's not kindness; that's insensitivity. Vegans also ration their compassion when they say, "I'm not going to have compassion for slaughterhouse workers, animal farmers, animal abusers, hunters, people who test on animals, people who eat animals, and [fill-in-the-blank] because they don't *deserve* my compassion." They use righteousness and—ironically—*compassion* as justification for their intolerance, forgetting that the people we think are the least deserving of our compassion are probably the ones who need it most.

> *Less* compassion in the world just means *less* compassion in the world. *More* compassion in the world means *more* compassion in the world.

If someone violates, hurts, or kills someone else—human or nonhuman—it's an indication that they're lacking compassion, empathy, awareness, or consciousness. The solution is not to withhold the very thing that's missing (compassion, empathy, awareness, consciousness) but to *fill* the lack with that thing. It doesn't matter *who* fills the void; what matters is that the void is filled. *Less* compassion in the world just means *less* compassion in the world. *More* compassion in the world means *more* compassion in the world. It really is that simple.

## 2. Highly effective advocates plant seeds and remain unattached to whether or not those seeds germinate.

As advocates who are desperate to end animal suffering, we think that if we provide enough information, show enough films, post enough social media photos, and say enough of the right things, people will become vegan, just as we did. I hear a lot of vegans say—with a little indignation in their voice—"I saw that film/heard that talk/read that book and became vegan overnight. How can someone see the same thing and *not* become vegan?!" We forget the dozens of other seeds planted along the way in our own journey leading up to the moment when we saw that movie or read that book. Perhaps it was the fifteenth seed that finally compelled us to do something different—to *become vegan*—or perhaps it was the 150th. The moment of awakening itself is often characterized as coming from out of the blue—"I became vegan overnight"—but with a little retrospection, most people would acknowledge that cracks had been visible prior to that moment—that "becoming vegan overnight" is really the culmination of years of fissures appearing in the foundation, enough that the walls can no longer hold.

When we present information to someone else and they *don't* become vegan, it isn't because we failed or because they're unfeeling; it may be because it's only the second seed planted for them or that the seeds that have been planted aren't ready to grow yet. There is no way to know, but that is no reason to despair. It's a reason to *keep planting seeds* and to keep watering them. We don't know what will be the final thing that compels someone to make a change, and in a way it's really not our business. Highly effective advocates plant seeds but remain unattached to *whether* or *when* those seeds will germinate.

Highly effective advocates also know when to stop overwatering the seeds they plant. I hear from a lot of advocates who say, "I've been trying to convince my uncle (or friend or family member) for five years that being vegan is healthier/better than eating meat, but he just argues. What can I say to persuade him?" My response? Move on! There are plenty of people who may want to hear what you have to say, but they're not hearing it because you're spending your time arguing with your uncle instead. Step back, let go, and when your uncle is interested, I bet he knows where he can find you if he wants more information. (In fact, when you stop pestering him, he may be more inclined to hear what you have to say.)

It may surprise you to learn that as someone who advocates for animals and compassion, my mission isn't "to make the world vegan" or "to change people's minds." If those were my goals, by all accounts I would be a failure as an advocate (and a pretty miserable person to boot). I would be a failure because I can't *make* anyone do anything. All I can do is speak the truth and trust that the truth will inspire others to act on their own values. While there are indeed effective and ineffective ways to advocate, human beings aren't a math equation to be solved. We are complex, psychological, habit-driven beings who resist change and abhor discomfort. For many people, willful blindness resolves the dissonance and discomfort they feel about their participation in animal cruelty or unhealthy eating habits. When they do the quick calculation in their minds, they see very little value in making behavioral changes that would disrupt how they eat, how they shop, how they socialize, and how they live. For those reasons and more, advocates have a tough hill to climb, and we need to understand the difference between leading and forcing. That is why I'm clear about my mission, which is *to empower people to make informed food choices, to raise awareness about violence against animals, and to give people the tools and resources they need to live according to their own values of compassion and wellness.* I'm very clear about those goals, and I can say unequivocally that I attain those goals every single day.

I believe we're here to be teachers for one another, and I'm grateful for my role as a conduit. But that's all any of us are. I don't take the credit for people becoming vegan from my work—just as I don't take the blame for people who don't become vegan despite my work. *Do your work, then step back*, says the *Tao Te Ching*. *The only path to serenity.*

### 3. Highly effective advocates never forget their own story.

It's imperative for those of us who have already become awake to remember where we came from—to remember that we, too, were once asleep and unaware. Perhaps we made stupid jokes, said silly things, defended our behavior. Perhaps we said, "I'll never be vegan"; perhaps we made fun of vegans. The point is, if we remember our story, we'll be less inclined to be self-righteous when we encounter people who are not where we're at. In forgetting our own stories, we lose our humility, and in doing so we risk becoming arrogant and self-righteous—not a great formula for remaining joyful or attracting people to this way of life. *Highly effective advocates know we're no better than anyone else for being vegan; we're just better today than we were yesterday.*

### 4. Highly effective advocates recognize there is more than one way to advocate.

Advocacy is not algebra. There isn't one single answer to the problems of animal cruelty, exploitation, and consumption. Although I do think some forms of advocacy are more effective than others, and I do think some methods turn other people off more than they draw them in, no single type of advocacy works best, because no single type works independent of the others. Individual forms of advocacy don't exist in a vacuum. It's not enough, for instance, to show people *why* they should be vegan; we also need to show them *how* to become vegan, and for that we need all the advocates who create the tools and resources that guide people through the transition.

We need advocates who create recipes, write books, make films, teach cooking classes, provide accurate nutrition information, and demystify vegan eating, cooking, living, and shopping. We also need innovators who create vegan products, investors who infuse money into these products, and lobbyists and trade groups who can ensure these products are equitably represented in the marketplace. We need advocates who raise awareness, write letters, screen documentaries, rescue animals, and run shelters and sanctuaries. We need advocates who help enact and enforce laws, change policies, educate, litigate, and legislate. We need advocates who change hearts and minds and those who change institutions such as schools, restaurants, corporations, and governments. We need it all. The animals need it all.

Whatever you choose to do, do it well, and know that you're making a difference. Whatever you choose *not* to do, get out of the way and let others do the work they have chosen. Just as all religions believe that God is on their side, so too can activists fall into the trap that they know exactly what works and that everyone else is wrong. Be wary of any activist who says that their single form of activism is the right way, and everyone else is hurting "the cause" rather than helping it. It's one thing to come together as fellow advocates to discuss efficacy, strategy, and improvements; it's quite another to devote precious time and to spend limited social capital publicly criticizing, condemning, and undermining other advocates—whether they're individuals or organizations. There are a lot of problems in this world, and there

> Worry less about people who don't agree with you. Harness instead the power and energy of the people who do agree with you, get to work, and let others do theirs.

are a lot of people who sit on their duffs doing absolutely nothing to solve them. There are fewer people who actually get up, speak out, and do something to make this world a better place. Advocates—even those with whom you disagree—who dedicate their time, resources, and money to help (animals *or* people) are *not the problem*. Apathy is the problem. In other words, worry less about people who don't agree with you. Harness instead the power and energy of the people who do agree with you, go do your work, and let others do theirs.

When my first book—*The Joy of Vegan Baking*—was published, I realized very quickly that I had to develop a thick skin if I was going to put my work out in the world. Everyone's a critic, of course, and with the prevalence of social media and websites that invite reviews, everyone has a public platform for voicing their criticism. I don't expect everyone to love everything I do, but what struck me were the "reviews" from people who promptly panned *The Joy of Vegan Baking* not because the writing, photographs, or recipes lacked merit but because it wasn't the book *they* wanted written—ostensibly one with recipes free of sugar, gluten, and oil. Clearly, my book wasn't a fit for them, but instead of just not buying the book, looking around for another, or writing their own, they took the time to excoriate mine and encourage others not to buy it.

Do your work, then step back. Everyone has a contribution to make—even if it's not the same as yours.

## 5. Highly effective advocates find common ground and build coalitions on that ground.

Effective advocates identify shared values, whether they are talking to their compatriots or advocating to nonvegans. They find common ground with people who may on the face of it seem like "the enemy" or "the opposition" and build from that common ground, standing together against violence rather than standing against one another—a great strategy for dealing with disagreement in any relationship about any issue. This is not always easy to do because you have to be more *willing to find resolution* than you are *eager to be right*; you have to be more willing to *solve the problem* than you are anxious to *win the argument.* Highly effective advocates ask, *Do I want to be right or do I want to be effective?*

> Highly effective advocates ask, *Do I want to be right or do I want to be effective?*

When it comes to talking to nonvegans, highly effective advocates know that people are surprised (and relieved) to know that vegans had a pre-vegan life. When someone says "I love meat" or "I could never give up cheese," they don't expect a vegan to say, "I did, too. I loved meat. I didn't stop eating meat because I stopped liking the taste; I stopped eating it because I realized it was made of animals" (or whatever is true for you). By doing so, not only will you be finding common ground with people, you will also be remembering and reinforcing your own story. It's incredibly effective (and incredibly kind) to acknowledge that you had a similar experience:

- ◆ "I used to think the same thing."
- ◆ "I totally understand."
- ◆ "I can absolutely relate."
- ◆ "I also grew up eating animals. I also thought it was going to be hard to stop."
- ◆ "I also never thought I could give up cheese."

If people find ways to identify with you, they'll be more inclined to consider making changes themselves or at least be open to hearing what you have to say. It's easy to stereotype someone we perceive as different from us and put them in a neat little box labeled NOT ME, presuming we know everything about them because of the category or categories we've placed them in. If you identify as a liberal, progressive, vegan, atheist Democrat, you may see anyone who is a conservative, religious,

Republican meat-eater as antithetical to you, and yet I'd wager that you have some things in common—even things you would agree on. Perhaps you both have dogs, cats, or children. Perhaps you both hate broccoli or love blueberry pancakes. Perhaps you both like hiking or chocolate or beer, or you both agree that animals shouldn't be victims of violence. There is always *something*, and I suggest you find it and start there. Rather than determine that you can't talk to someone about a sensitive subject because you have such different viewpoints, try to have a more catholic perspective that appreciates the common ground you share and that respects the common ground you don't. This applies broadly as well, whether you're creating coalitions with other movements, working with opposing political parties on nonpartisan legislation, or finding common ground with other animal and vegan advocates and organizations. Effective advocates know they don't need to agree with others about *everything* in order to work together on *something*.

## 6. Highly effective advocates understand that perfection is the enemy of the good.

"This is Earth. It will never be heaven. There will always be cruelty, always be violence, always be destruction. We cannot eliminate all devastation for all time, but we can reduce it, outlaw it, undermine its sources and foundations: these are victories. A better world, yes; a perfect world, never."[3] These are the words of the brilliant activist Rebecca Solnit from her small gem of a book, *Hope in the Dark,* which celebrates activism as a journey rather than as a means for achieving Utopia. Similarly, in his book *Enlightenment Now,* cognitive psychologist Steven Pinker makes the case that in every way progress can be measured (health, prosperity, safety, peace, knowledge, happiness), things are better now than they used to be, even though there is still much work to be done. But not everyone wants to believe in progress—especially, it seems, progressives. "There's a tendency among intellectuals to point to every unsolved problem as the symptom of a sick society,"[4] says Pinker; like Solnit, he reminds us that although we will never have a perfect world, that doesn't mean we should stop trying to make it better.

Both authors challenge a view cherished mostly by progressives that we can't talk about any good things until there are no more bad things and that we can't celebrate progress until everything is perfect. Some animal advocates succumb to this manner of thinking when they criticize instead of celebrate any incremental progress toward the larger goal of eliminating systemic violence against animals:

- They disparage campaigns, such as Meatless Monday, that encourage people to eat *less* meat, dairy, and eggs or any program that helps people transition over a period of time, such as the 30-Day Vegan Challenge or Veganuary.
- They call for boycotts of vegan products whose manufacturers receive investments from nonvegan companies for the purpose of increasing the availability and affordability of vegan products in the marketplace.
- They oppose any welfare laws that make it illegal to confine, mutilate, and mistreat animals used for food, entertainment, fur, or research.

They characterize any type of advocacy other than that which tells people to "go vegan" as a betrayal to the animals.

Let me tell you a little story.

At the end of 2014, an ordinance to ban the use of bullhooks on elephants was brought before the Oakland City Council. Bullhooks are sharp weapons used to hurt and intimidate elephants to force them to perform unnatural acts for the amusement of humans. Some advocates decried the ordinance, saying that it was just a welfare measure and that if we really wanted to make a difference for animals, we should ask the city council to ban the circus altogether. Feld Entertainment, the owner of Ringling Bros. Circus, showed up with expensive lawyers and spent a lot of money in Oakland (and previously in Los Angeles) to fight the bull-hook ban. They lost. As cities and counties across the United States began drafting legislation similar to that which passed in Oakland (and before that in Los Angeles), Ringling recognized how expensive it would be to fight in small local jurisdictions across the nation. They also knew that without bullhooks, they wouldn't be able to train (read: torture) these large, sensitive, social animals—and so they made the announcement that they were removing elephant acts from all of their circuses.

It was a victory to be sure, but many advocates lamented the fate of the other circus victims—the tigers, lions, and bears. *What's the difference if other animals are still suffering? What we really need to do is close the circus!* Except the story wasn't over. Without elephant acts, the circus's main moneymaker, Ringling couldn't attract enough audience members to remain profitable, and in May 2017, after 146 years, Ringling Brothers and Barnum & Bailey closed for good. A ban on a single weapon used on a single species triggered the demise of the most famous of American circuses—an incremental step that broke the circus's back.

Most advocates celebrated the victory, but some blamed other activists for not ensuring that all of Ringling's animals would go to sanctuaries. "Perfectionists can find fault with anything," writes Solnit. "Perfectionists hold that anything less than total victory is failure, a premise that makes it easy to give up at the start or to disparage the victories that are possible."[5] We have no idea the impact our activism will have, and none of us can predict the outcome. Highly effective advocates do the best they can, let others do the work they do, celebrate victories, and don't let perfectionism be a stick with which to beat the possible.

Health-food vegan advocates can also let their vision of a perfect world hinder progress when they insist that anything short of a whole-foods, unprocessed, sugar-free, gluten-free, oil-free, plant-based diet is unhealthy. They rail against the very existence of vegan meats, cheeses, and other convenience foods, claiming they're as unhealthy as animal-based versions. They attack those they dub "junk-food vegans" and censure cookbook authors and food bloggers for using oil, flour, sugar, or any other ingredient they deem unfit for human consumption in their recipes. The fact is, everything and everyone is on a spectrum, and we have to meet people where they're at. It's rare—and difficult—for someone to go from eating fat-laden steaks and greasy French fries every day to basing their diet on sweet potatoes and kale. Many of the more highly processed foods help people transition from their meat-, dairy-, and egg-based habits, and despite claims to the contrary, measure for measure, vegan meats, dairy-free cheeses, and other vegan foods in the marketplace are loads healthier than animal products. Admittedly, that's a low bar to begin with, but that's the point. It's all relative. A bowl of pinto beans is more nutrient-dense than a Beyond Burger, but a Beyond Burger is healthier than a beef burger.

Technically speaking, the term "processed" refers to any food that has been washed, cleaned, cut, milled, chopped, heated, pasteurized, blanched, boiled, cooked, canned, jarred, frozen, mixed, blended, or packaged; in other words, any food that is in any way altered from its whole natural state could be considered a "processed food." The orange juice you squeeze into a glass from a fresh orange is *processed*. The fresh blueberries you blend into a smoothie are *processed*. The fresh tomatoes your grandmother taught you to can and the fresh kale you dehydrate are both technically *processed* foods. Eating foods in their different states brings pleasure and variety to our lives; there's a reason one of our favorite kitchen appliances is called a *food processor*.

Instead of disparaging "processed foods" as a monolith, we can make a distinction between minimally processed and highly processed foods and recognize that even the latter have their place. Considering how easy the meat, dairy, and egg industries make it for people to eat unhealthy animal products, we should be grateful that people can choose meat-, dairy-, and egg-free items in the marketplace. Aspiring to make whole foods the foundation of our diet means doing the best we can—not striving for perfection—and creating a space for others to do the same.

## 7. Highly effective advocates are committed to self-care.

Many advocates suffer from the mistaken assumption that self-care is egocentric, but in fact, the opposite is true. The consequences of not attending to our physical, mental, emotional, social, spiritual, and financial needs can be dire and detrimental to our efficacy as advocates and to our health as human beings. We can suffer from empathic distress (see Stage One), anger (see Stage Five), rage, self-righteousness, cynicism, low self-esteem, fatigue, depression, ill health, debt, unemployment, or burnout. Make no mistake about it: self-care isn't selfish, it's sensible; it's not self-indulgent, it's self-preservation. Your activism isn't lessened by self-care; it thrives by it, and the recipients of your activism—whether human or animal—are better served when you commit to it.

Highly effective advocates know they don't have to suffer in order to be effective, and in fact are less effective when they are suffering. They know when their resources are running low so they can replenish them before they're fully depleted, and they recognize the value of investing in self-care—a broad term that really just means being as compassionate with yourself as you would be with others you care about. Practicing daily self-care is a sure-fire way to not only keep your tank full, but even have some reserves when you're having a particularly difficult day, and it's the most effective way to prevent burnout. You can't give what you don't have. The benefits of self-care are manifold, including more resilience, improved resistance to disease, enhanced self-esteem, and increased self-knowledge.

Creating a self-care plan doesn't take much time, but whatever time you do invest will come back to you tenfold. Customize your own plan based on what your values are and on what you genuinely enjoy. Here are a few suggestions:

→  Eat well.
→  Cry when compelled.

→ Laugh.

→ Spend time in nature.

→ Exercise.

→ Get sufficient sleep.

→ Surround yourself with supportive, compassionate people.

→ Find quiet time.

→ Disengage from social media.

→ Implement periodic news blackouts.

→ Read a book unrelated to animal rights or veganism.

→ Give yourself a break from activism. Activist guilt is a real thing; give yourself permission to say *no*.

→ Drink tea.

→ Spend time with animals.

→ Tend to financial needs.

→ Practice mindfulness (see page 81 for the Loving-Kindness Meditation).

→ Express gratitude. Numerous recent studies have found that people who write down or even consciously think about what they're grateful for tend to be happier and less depressed.[6]

Prioritizing self-care in all aspects of our lives will make us better advocates and can even provide a model for others who struggle with self-care to follow.

## 8. Highly effective advocates know their message, stay on message, and repeat their message.

If you asked vegan advocates what their primary message is, the majority of them would most likely say that it's "Go vegan" or "It's wrong/cruel/unhealthy to eat animals." What I'm encouraging you to do is get even clearer than that. For instance, here's my basic message:

*Animals are here for their own purposes and not for our use. Animals don't exist to be our entertainment, our food, our test subjects, or our shooting targets. They have value completely separate from humans. We are part of their community, and they are part of ours, as residents, co-inhabitants, and contributors; they are not outsiders or intruders. My message is that to use violence against nonhuman animals is to perpetuate violence against ourselves and one another. My message is that we are all connected. My message is compassion.*

Everything I say or write reflects my message, my worldview. Take the time to clarify your own. Once you've done so, share it—then repeat it. When we repeat our message, we strengthen it. Although many of the new people in your circle of influence will be hearing it for the first time, those hearing it for the thousandth time will have it reinforced in their brains.

So, know your message, repeat your message, and then *stay on message*. It's easy to get distracted and reactive, or to be persuaded by other advocates who think *your* message should reflect *their* message. Resist the temptation. Finding a good, effective message and then sticking with it takes extraordinary discipline, but it pays off in the end. It keeps you focused, and it makes your message very clear to others—who can then repeat it to even more people.

Finally, advocates who use "Go vegan" as their mantra may want to consider the research that shows that people respond better to the language of *values* than *ideology*.[7] And to most people, veganism is not a value. It's a *manifestation* of values (kindness, simplicity, responsibility, self-care), but it's not a *value* in people's minds. In fact, most people perceive it as an *ideology*. In other words, when advocates exclaim "Go vegan!" they're not really speaking to a value or identity that has the potential to resonate with people. What's more, treating veganism as an identity that people should adopt usually backfires, because many people associate veganism as being antithetical to their existing identities, as we discussed in Stage Six. So if we're thinking strategically as advocates, then the message we communicate cannot simply be "Go vegan," because to most people, "vegan" is just an ideology, and adhering to an ideology is not a moral, or values-based, goal for people. *Being a good person* is a moral goal. *Being kind* is a moral goal. *Not hurting anyone* is a moral goal. So, break down "veganism" into the language of *values* and *morals* instead. Frame your message in terms of moral goals such

> To most people, veganism is not a value. It's a *manifestation* of values.

as compassion, justice, kindness, protection, simplicity, nonviolence, wellness, nonharm, and integrity, and you will be much more effective.

## 9. Highly effective advocates have perspective and vision. They learn from the past, stand firmly in the present, and keep their eye on the future.

As human beings and as ambassadors of compassion, we need to know on whose shoulders we stand not only to fully appreciate the importance of this work but also to understand that we are part of something very old and very profound. Therefore, highly effective advocates seek to learn about the advocates who came before them, whose courage and conviction shaped the vegan and animal protection movements as we know them today. It is their mistakes we can learn from and their successes we can emulate. Our movement has an incredible history, and yet it is virtually unknown. If vegan and animal advocates don't know the history of our cause, we have no sense of our movement's struggles, long-term strategies, achievements, and heroes. What's more, if we don't know and thus don't promote our long, impressive history to the public, then opponents of the movements will fill the void by constructing their own false story.

For example, by promoting the history of animal protection, advocates could smash the myth that we are misanthropes; history shows this to be patently false since most early animal advocates were involved in multiple social justice movements, and many still are today. This unfounded dichotomy often cited between animal rights and human rights comes directly from the opponents of the animal protection movement, who have done a better job than animal advocates of controlling the story, the history, and the perceptions of animal advocacy. If animal advocates not only learned their history, but also made it part of their mission to get that history out to the public, I believe it would greatly benefit the movement overall. We would be better able to speak to the fact that many of the early founders of the animal protection movement in the UK and in the US were active in other social justice areas: in the abolition of slavery, in the suffrage movement, in peace movements. See the sidebar on page 260 for some examples of this.

We need to dispel the myth that work on behalf of animals hinders humanitarian issues. In fact, with all the in-fighting about the word *vegan*, advocates would do well to understand that early animal advocates actually called themselves "humanitarians." These were people who were challenging the very bedrock of human superiority, but one of their goals was also to make *human* society more moral and humane, thus they considered themselves *humanitarians*, in the sense that stopping cruelty was also about bettering *humanity*. They also referred to themselves as protectionists, humane agents, zoophilists, rightists, and welfarists. If you want to immerse yourself in the history of the animal protection movement, I recommend starting with Kathryn Shevelow's book *For the Love of Animals: The Rise of the Animal Protection Movement*, whose focus is on its inception in the United Kingdom, and Diane Beers's book, *For the Prevention of Cruelty: The History and Legacy of Animal Rights Activism in the United States*, which documents the history of the animal protection movement in the United States. As for the history of vegetarianism and veganism, I recommend *The Bloodless Revolution: A Cultural History of Vegetarianism from 1600 to Modern Times* by Tristram Stuart, *The Heretic's Feast: A History of Vegetarianism* by Colin Spencer, and *Vegetarian America: A History* by Karen Iacobbo and Michael Iacobbo.

Learning about our past is also crucial to having perspective in the present. Both historically and recently, divisions in the movement have threatened and even undermined potentially successful campaigns. There is nothing new about that, nor is it unique to the animal protection movement or the vegan movement, but these divisions are an important measure of a movement's health and success. Internal ideological or strategic differences can invigorate a movement with new ideas and energy, but they can also tear it apart, and there is much we can learn from our past about how to manage them. Different opinions and ideas should not be silenced, but one of the questions organizations and individual advocates need to ask themselves is how a movement can best embrace them.

> Learning about our past is crucial to having perspective in the present.

Finally, as much as we need to look to the past, we also need to be rooted in the present, while planning for the future. One of the ways to sustain our activism is to recognize that we're in this for the long haul—that animal advocacy is a marathon, not a sprint. We've come a long way, but we still have far to go, and in order to carry on as a movement, we need to build the future brick by brick. If you focus only on individual bricks, with all of their messy mortar, you begin to feel you're making no progress at all. If you instead step back, acknowledge your progress, and commit to the big picture, you'll wipe your brow, take a breath, and get back to stacking those bricks.

## 10. Highly effective advocates have hope.

I talk about hope as an antidote to anger in Stage Five, but because hope is also part of the formula for effective advocacy, it needs to be mentioned here as well. Highly effective advocates have hope because there is much to be hopeful about:

- The concept of veganism—living compassionately and healthfully—is more mainstream than ever before.

- More people are speaking up on behalf of animals and plant-based eating than ever before.

- Animal-free meats, cheeses, and milks are available in grocery stores and in restaurants all around the world, and those options are only increasing.

- Animal-based meat and milk companies see the writing on the wall and are creating their own plant-based products or investing in those that have proven successful.

- Scientific advances and technological breakthroughs such as cellular agriculture, GPS tracking, and drone technologies have the potential to save billions of animals from poaching, factory farming, and systemic abuse.

- Visionaries are creating innovative products—for animal-free food, clothing, and materials—that increase our choices in the marketplace and enable us to support companies and products that reflect our taste and ethics, while rejecting those that don't.

- For those of us who live in democracies—and the majority of countries are democratic[8]—we can criticize elected officials, vote them out, and exercise our power and privilege to help those who have neither, including animals.

- More and more countries are banning circuses that have animal acts.

- Animal welfare is now taken seriously as a legislative issue.

Highly effective advocates are messengers of hope rather than of doom—not only because there is reason to hope but also because a steady stream of crisis-messaging depletes people's will and ability to engage with social problems. While framing everything as a crisis or a catastrophe might generate clicks on social media, the emotions they inspire tend to be either fleeting or fatalistic, leaving people feeling that social problems are overwhelming and unsolvable and causing them to turn away with a sense of frustration and help-lessness. As advocates, we tend to focus a lot on problems, but it should be no surprise that people are pretty clear about the prob-lems. We need to do a better job focusing on the solutions, and on painting them as vividly and con-

> Highly effective advocates are messengers of hope rather than messengers of doom.

cretely as we do the problems—that is, more specifically and tangibly than just saying "Go vegan." So, while we need to alert people to the problems animals face, we need even more to alert them to the problems we can all solve.

In her book *Hope in the Dark*, Rebecca Solnit channels her philosophy of hope through the words of Virginia Woolf, who wrote in her diary in 1915: "The future is dark, which is the best thing the future can be, I think." It's tempting to interpret darkness as dismal and dreary, but Solnit reframes it: "Most people are afraid of the dark. . . . Many adults fear, above all, the darkness that is the unknown, the unseeable, the obscure. And yet the night in which distinctions and definitions cannot be readily made is the same night in which love is made, in which things merge, change, become enchanted, aroused, impregnated, possessed, released, renewed."[9] In other words, the future isn't dark because it's bleak; it's dark because it's inscrutable. It's inscrutable because it has not yet been written. So go write it. Go write the future today.

# Historical Humanitarians

Here are just a few examples of how the struggle against animal abuse and exploitation has always been bound up in other social justice issues and how early activists advocated for many of them across the board. Believing that stopping cruelty against animals also benefits humanity, some early animal advocates called themselves *humanitarians*, and many founders of the animal protection movement in the UK and in the US were active in other social justice areas.

**William Wilberforce:** A British politician, philanthropist, and Member of Parliament from 1780 to 1825, Wilberforce was the first to introduce a bill to abolish the slave trade; he opposed slavery on ethical grounds and was also a voice for animals. He was active in educational reform, prison reform, the promotion of public health initiatives, and advocating for better working conditions for factory workers. As an extension of his concern for justice, in 1824 he helped found the Royal Society for the Prevention of Cruelty to Animals, which is the predecessor of the American Society for the Prevention of Cruelty to Animals.

**Henry Bergh:** Believing that "mercy to animals means mercy to mankind," Bergh was the first to successfully challenge the prevailing view that both animals and children were property with no rights of their own. He founded the American Society for the Prevention of Cruelty to Animals in 1866 and cofounded the New York Society for the Prevention of Cruelty to Children in 1875.

**Caroline Earle White:** An American philanthropist and tireless activist, White worked on behalf of the suffrage movement and the abolition of slavery, and in 1867 cofounded the Philadelphia Society for the Prevention of Cruelty to Animals, which became the American Anti-Vivisection Society, an organization still thriving and succeeding today on behalf of animals.

**Henry Salt:** A British writer and literary critic born in 1851, Salt is credited as the first writer to advocate for animal *rights* (rather than just improving their *welfare*). Salt formed the Humanitarian League in 1891 with the aim of banning hunting as a sport; in addition to dedicating his life to animal advocacy, he was also actively involved in other social justice areas, such as the reform of prisons, criminal justice, and schools.

**George Thorndike Angell:** An American lawyer and philanthropist, Angell founded the Massachusetts Society for the Prevention of Cruelty to Animals in 1868, and in 1889 founded the American Humane Education Society. Dedicating his life to the humane treatment of animals, he also crusaded for humans, advocating for public health and against the adulteration of food.

# Integration and Adaptation

## Identifying as a Joyful Vegan in a Nonvegan World

*The art of life lies in a constant readjustment to our surroundings.*
—Kakuzō Okakura, *The Book of Tea*

Whereas the previous chapter is all about how we can contribute to creating a vegan world, this chapter is all about how veganism now fits into our world. At this stage in our journey, being vegan is just part of who we are. What might have felt like an effort when we first transitioned is now a natural, normal aspect of our lives. What might have once felt like a struggle now feels like a joy. Our friends and family have acclimated to our changes—some may have even joined us—and meals are no longer laden with tension. We ask for what we need without fear or stress, and we find that people are happy to accommodate us without hassle or irritation. At this stage, we embrace the fact that in order to make a difference, we may have to do something different, but *different* doesn't mean *inferior*—and neither does it mean *superior*. We know we're no better than anyone else for being vegan; we're just better than we were yesterday and the day before that.

> We know we're no better than anyone else for being vegan; we're just better than we were yesterday and the day before that.

When veganism is fully integrated into our lives, we consider it a victory when we find one vegan item out of twenty on a restaurant menu—and a triumph when we see that ten of those twenty items could be easily veganized with just a small tweak. When veganism is fully integrated into our lives, we feel elated when our workmates ask us for vegan recipes and our neighbors include vegan dishes at the annual summer fête. Or when our special meal at a wedding inspires envy in all the other guests. We celebrate when we travel to meat-laden countries and see vegan options in the unlikeliest of places; we may not find a five-star gourmet vegan restaurant, but we're thankful for and make the most of what we do find. It's not that our expectations are low; it's that we see abundance rather than limitation, plenty rather than scarcity. We feel grateful rather than entitled, and we embrace the lifestyle we have chosen: aspiring to live with integrity and compassion, knowing that every decision we make is done with the intention of not contributing to the suffering and exploitation of human and nonhuman animals and of not causing harm to ourselves. We accept that we will make mistakes, because we know our goal is not perfection. Our goal is to strive for unconditional compassion and optimal wellness, and we see veganism as a tool for achieving these goals. Embracing our vegan identity means embracing the journey and welcoming its imperfections—being adaptive, creative, flexible, humble, truthful, playful, patient, emotional, unapologetic, and fully human with all our flaws and foibles.

# THE NEW NORMAL

The anecdotal and empirical accounts of improved emotional, mental, and physical health among vegetarians and vegans are vast and well documented. Aside from the measurable and observable physical changes that take place—improved cholesterol, increased energy, decreased weight, improved digestion and regularity, improved kidney function, decreased arthritic pain—when veganism is integrated into your life, there are a number of other things you become accustomed to and amused by, things that become the new normal.

- **The vegan jokes will persist.** Most likely you will be subjected to the same comments twenty years from now as you are today. You can shrug, roll your eyes, politely ask that they stop, and even laugh—and know that the next one is just around the corner.

- **People will always suffer from *whataboutism*.** As a matter of self-preservation, people will deflect the harm of their own actions by trying to discredit veganism and by pointing out the supposed hypocrisy of those who identify as vegan:

  — *You're vegan? Well, what about plants? They have feelings, too!*
  — *You're vegan? Well, what about the fake leather you wear? That's environmentally destructive!*
  — *You're vegan? Well, what about the insects you kill when you drive your car? That's not very compassionate!*

  Some of these questions are asked out of genuine curiosity and some are asked to try and catch you in some logical flaw that will justify meat, dairy, and egg consumption and undermine this compassionate and healthful way of living. I often joke that people expect vegans to have advanced degrees in nutrition, philosophy, history, anthropology, religion, animal husbandry, ecology, and the culinary arts—and it's only funny because it's true. Feel free to respond to such questions—applying the strategies discussed in Stage Seven on communication—but just don't be surprised when you hear them again and again.

- **Everyone is an expert.** While no one cared about your increased risk for heart disease while when you were shoving meat, cheese, and eggs in your mouth, suddenly everybody is a self-declared dietitian when they hear about your veganism. Get used to it.

- **Everyone wants to know what you eat.** Everyone, from complete strangers to close family members, is curious about what you eat—because they really don't know. *You* may know you don't eat iceberg lettuce every day, but *they* may not. *You* may know how easy it is to bake without eggs, but *they* may not. I'm not suggesting you have to entertain every question you're asked, but they are part of the territory, and they're wonderful opportunities to debunk some myths about what it means to be vegan.

- **Some friends and family will fuss over your veganism—in a good way.** Some of your loved ones—even just casual friends or coworkers—will be very protective of you, going out of their way to make sure you have something to eat at an event you're attending together or calling a restaurant ahead of time to find out what's vegan. You may feel like much ado is being made unnecessarily, but just appreciate the support.

- **You don't know everything.** And that's okay. You know when I said there's an expectation that vegans have advanced degrees in nutrition, philosophy, history, anthropology, religion, animal husbandry, ecology, and the culinary arts? Well, that expectation doesn't come only from nonvegans; it may come from you as well.

We put so much pressure on ourselves to have the perfect answer to every question we're asked, but here's something to get used to: you don't know everything, and you don't have to. You can say, "I don't know," and the world will still turn. As much as you've learned, there is always something you haven't yet. Just remain humble and open to new thoughts, ideas, and perspectives.

## WHAT MAY SURPRISE YOU

◆ **Your food awareness increases**—not just in terms of ingredients and cuisines that become familiar to you but in terms of being more mindful about what and how you're eating. Whether you become vegan for health reasons or not, as time goes on, you do tend to seek out more nutrient-dense foods.

◆ **You have more impact on people than you realize.** While I encourage you to keep your expectations in check, you will discover that you've inspired some people to make changes in the way they eat just because they see your changes. They may not have become vegan, but they may have swapped some nonvegan products for vegan ones and they cook more vegan dishes than they did before you become vegan. That's something to celebrate.

◆ **You become more tolerant**. The passion that fueled you in your early days continues to burn but with a little less heat. You accept that some of your family and friends may never become vegan, but you love them all the same.

◆ **You wear vegan messagewear.** Although you never thought you'd wear your veganism on your sleeve, you do so now—literally—on shirts, baseball caps, tote bags, and even tattoos.

◆ **You decide to keep a vegan home—but you compromise when necessary.** In the beginning you thought you could handle having animal products cooked or brought into your home, but now you just want one little corner of the world where the sights and smells of animal products don't penetrate. Of course, if you live with roommates or loved ones who do eat animal products, it's important to find a way to meet everyone's needs. Compromise is key. See the sidebar on page 131 for suggestions.

- **You date nonvegans.** You realize that if you set out to find a match only among vegans, your pool would be very small, so you broaden your criteria by searching not specifically for "someone who is vegan" but for "someone who is loving, kind, intelligent, compassionate, and thoughtful."

- **You know that being vegan is not a panacea, but it's still the best road you've found to living as compassionately and healthfully as possible.** You let your actions and values speak for themselves and don't feel you have to be a perfect poster child for veganism. You may get sick, make mistakes, and gain/lose weight—whether you're vegan or not. You may have love handles, drink too much, get overly emotional, and succumb to your worst character defects. By being the best vegan you can be, you will remain *human*—flawed, imperfect, vulnerable to illness, and destined for death.

When veganism is fully integrated into our lives, the conscious choices we make feel liberating rather than limiting, and we accept that reading labels, constantly being asked about veganism, and having fewer menu options in restaurants are small prices to pay for the potential to manifest our deepest values in our everyday behavior. Where others may see lack, we see possibility; where others may see inconvenience, we see opportunity. There are many reasons people think being vegan is about restriction rather than expansion, and I think it has to do with the perception that being vegan is about saying no—about *refusing* things that are offered to us. It *appears* that being vegan is about denial and sacrifice, and that's the problem—the *perception* of what it means to live vegan. If you're on the outside looking in, you tend to see only what vegans *don't* choose. You don't see what we *are* choosing. In public settings in a world dominated by the animal-eating culture, people see vegans rejecting things far more than they see them embracing things. And that's the gift. That's the surprise. Though being vegan does involve saying no to some things—namely *unhealthy foods, destructive environmental practices, animal cruelty,* and *egregious violence*—at its core, being vegan is about saying yes.

> By choosing to eat life-giving rather than life-taking foods, we're saying "yes" to our values of wellness and health, of peace and nonviolence, of kindness and compassion.

By choosing to eat life-giving rather than life-taking foods, we're saying yes to our values of wellness and health, of peace and nonviolence, of kindness and compassion. By choosing to look at what we do to other animals for our convenience and pleasure, we're saying yes to our values of accountability, responsibility, and commitment to truth and knowledge. By standing up for our beliefs and speaking up on behalf of those who have no voice, we're saying yes to our values of justice, courage, and service to others. Being vegan is about saying yes to the bounty of plant-based options that are available to all of us. Being vegan is about saying yes to our values. What's the use in having values if we don't manifest them in our behavior? Being vegan, which extends to every area of our lives, is an opportunity to do just that: to put our abstract values into concrete action.

It's ironic, of course, that being vegan is perceived as restrictive, since the majority of people, including all of us before we were vegan, choose to live in willful blindness, closing our eyes and cuffing our ears, saying, *Don't tell me what happens to animals. I don't want to know. Don't tell me how unhealthy this hot dog is. I don't want to hear.* We quite explicitly *hinder* our awareness because we're afraid to look, afraid to know, afraid to change. To me, that's limiting. That's restrictive. On the contrary, being vegan is about being willing to know, willing to explore, willing to look, willing to experience what is painful but true.

To me that's expansive. That's abundance. That's vegan.

# WHEN ONE JOURNEY ENDS, ANOTHER BEGINS

In the fairy tales of our childhood, once the princess is awakened and she has her prince, the story ends. We're never told what happens next, but we imagine a utopian future of everlasting bliss and perpetual joy—although we know that's not what living looks like. In the late 1980s, a musical by Stephen Sondheim and James Lapine reimagined these stories for us and fashioned a more realistic and recognizable future. *Into the Woods* follows the familiar storylines from several Grimm fairy tales, including *Snow White* and *Sleeping Beauty*, but extends their plots to reveal that there is no "happily after ever." There's happiness and peace and contentment and relief, but there's also anxiety, anger, nostalgia, suspicion, remorse, denial, and dread. And so the journey continues, and so it will never end. But the characters are stronger for it and wiser and in the company of fellow seekers.

> Into the woods—you have to grope,
> But that's the way you learn to cope.
> Into the woods to find there's hope
> Of getting through the journey.

Ours, too, is a story with no ending, a journey with no destination. Savor the highlights, take note of the landmarks, and go up, through, or around the obstacles you will inevitably encounter. Travel above and beyond what's familiar, whether you go around the block or around the globe. If you've lived your whole life seeing the world from your front door, it might feel overwhelming, but it's worth it, and you're not alone. Many before you have traversed the same ground, and many will follow behind. Take this book with you, and may it be a map to guide you.

# ACKNOWLEDGMENTS

I want to thank:

Everyone who has ever written to me and shared your stories of transformation; your struggles, challenges, and pitfalls; and your joys, triumphs, and victories. Each and every letter I receive informs the work I do and impacts those who are touched by it.

My mom and dad for supporting me even when I wasn't so joyful.

My biggest champion, my husband David.

My furry little gifts, Charlie and Michiko.

My besties, Kristie, Melissa, Greg, and Tim.

My sisters and brothers, Kenda, Susie, Deb, Milena, Donna L., Donna F., Lori, Cathleen, Tim, Ellen, Diane, Amanda, Devin, Michael S., Michael C., and Alex.

My helpers and allies, Danielle, Raitis, Florian, Michelle, and Hannah.

My partners, Brighde and Seb.

My angels, Alex, David, and Morgan.

My editor, Leah, whose keen insight, perception, and sensitivity made *The Joyful Vegan* a better book.

My inspiration, the animals.

My teachers. (Yes, that means *you*.)

# SPECIAL RECOGNITION

I'm so grateful to the special individuals below who generously support my work as monthly patrons. On behalf of the animals, thank you for helping me help people manifest their values of compassion and wellness in their everyday lives.

Alexander Gray and David Cabrera

Anke Keilich

Ann Merrill

Bailey Manlosa

Becky Peters

Belen Melendrez

Boni Lamson

Brece Clark

Brooke Bussard

Brooke Hueper

Caroline Dyar

Cheri Brown

Cini Bretzlaff-Holstein

Cristina Fisher

Debra Knutson

Delfina Lopez

Geneviève Okuma

Gina Carr

Heather Elise Goodwin

Janet Ratliff

Janette Gilmour

Jayson Biggins

Jennifer Guerra

Jennifer Watkins

Jerilynn Hilmar

Johanna Veth

Jonathan Brant

Joseph Sailor

Kari Parker

Katariina Forsberg

Kenda English

Korshi Dosoo and Davide Galli

Kristin Beecraft

Laura Hastings

Laura Lichterman

Leana Lovejoy

Liv Larsen

Liz Dee

Lydia Ruth Huston

Lyndall Sargent

Marie-Eve Bedard

Matthew and Nina King

Max Goodman

Megan Lindeman

Melissa Amarello

Michael Rooney

Michal Stone

Michelle Mabe

Mike McNeeley

Morgan Hall

Nikki DeSarno

Nina Bircher

P. J. Schuster

Patricia Hagmann

Patrick Reilly

Paul Zhang

Ranjini Mohan

Rassmus Peterson

Roland Reid

Rosalie Black

Sandy Kraus Smith

Sara Dee

Sheri Mersola

Sue Ellis Dyar

Susan Kiger

Tammy Robertson

Thomas J. Baechle

Tim Anderson

Tina Strasheim

Todd Hilson

# RESOURCES AND RECOMMENDATIONS

## THE FIRST ANIMAL PROTECTION AND VEGAN BOOKS I READ

Sue Coe, *Dead Meat*

Brenda Davis and Vesanto Melina, *Becoming Vegan*

Gail Eisnitz, *Slaughterhouse: The Shocking Story of Greed, Neglect, and Inhumane Treatment Inside the U.S. Meat Industry*

Howard Lyman, *Mad Cowboy: Plain Truth from the Cattle Rancher Who Won't Eat Meat*

Jim Mason, *An Unnatural Order: Roots of Our Destruction of Nature*

Charles Patterson, *Eternal Treblinka: Our Treatment of Animals and the Holocaust*

Tom Regan, *The Case for Animal Rights*

John Robbins, *Diet for a New America*

Matthew Scully, *Dominion: The Power of Man, the Suffering of Animals, and the Call to Mercy*

Peter Singer, *Animal Liberation*

Peter Singer, *Ethics into Action: Henry Spira and the Animal Rights Movement*

Marjorie Spiegel, *The Dreaded Comparison: Human and Animal Slavery*

Steven M. Wise, *Rattling the Cage: Toward Legal Rights for Animals*

## THE FIRST COOKBOOKS I BOUGHT

Tanya Barnard and Sarah Kramer, *How It All Vegan*

Mari Fujii, *The Enlightened Kitchen*

Nicola Graimes, *The Vegan Cookbook*

Louise Hagler, *Tofu Cookery*

Donna Klein, *The Mediterranean Vegan Kitchen*

Donna Klein, *Vegan Italiano*

Judy Krizmanic, *The Teen's Vegetarian Cookbook*

Jennifer Raymond, *The Peaceful Palate*

Robin Robertson, *Vegan Planet*

Joanne Stepaniak, *Vegan Vittles*

Eric Tucker, *The Millennium Cookbook*

Susan Walter, *Vegetarian Cooking at the Academy*

## OTHER RECOMMENDED READING

I've included these books here because they have either shaped my thinking related to my work and life or because I think they may be helpful for you on your journey.

Jonathan Balcombe, *Second Nature: The Inner Lives of Animals*

Jonathan Balcombe, *What a Fish Knows: The Inner Lives of Our Underwater Cousins*

Diane Beers, *For the Prevention of Cruelty: The History and Legacy of Animal Rights Activism in the United States*

Marc Bekoff and Jessica Pierce, *Wild Justice: The Moral Lives of Animals*

Craig Childs, *The Animal Dialogues: Uncommon Encounters in the Wild*

Stanley Cohen, *States of Denial: Knowing About Atrocities and Suffering*

Stephanie Feldstein, *The Animal Lover's Guide to Changing the World*

Jonathan Safran Foer, *Eating Animals*

Ted Genoways, *The Chain: Farm, Factory, and the Fate of Our Food*

Maya Gottfried, *Vegan Love: Dating and Partnering for the Cruelty-Free Gal, with Fashion, Makeup, and Wedding Tips*

Yuval Noah Harari, *Sapiens: A Brief History of Humankind*

Mark Hawthorne, *Striking at the Roots: A Practical Guide to Animal Activism*

Margaret Heffernan, *Willful Blindness: Why We Ignore the Obvious at Our Peril*

Karen Iacobbo and Michael Iacobbo, *Vegetarian America: A History*

Melanie Joy, *Beyond Beliefs: A Guide to Improving Relationships and Communication for Vegans, Vegetarians, and Meat Eaters*

Melanie Joy, *Why We Love Dogs, Eat Pigs, and Wear Cows: An Introduction to Carnism*

Tobias Leenaert, *How to Create a Vegan World: A Pragmatic Approach*

Greg Lukianoff and Jonathan Haidt, *The Coddling of the American Mind: How Good Intentions and Bad Ideas Are Setting Up a Generation for Failure*

Stephen Mitchell (translator), *Bhagavad Gita*

Stephen Mitchell (translator), *Tao Te Ching*

George Monbiot, *Feral: Rewilding the Land, the Sea, and Human Life*

Sy Montgomery, *How to Be a Good Creature: A Memoir in Thirteen Animals*

Sy Montgomery, *The Good Good Pig: The Extraordinary Life of Christopher Hogwood*

Tai Moses, *Zooburbia: Meditations on the Wild Animals Among Us*

Lani Muelrath, *The Mindful Vegan: A 30-Day Plan for Finding Health, Balance, Peace, and Happiness*

Marion Nestle, *Food Politics: How the Food Industry Influences Nutrition and Health*

Richard Oppenlander, *Comfortably Unaware: Global Depletion and Food Responsibility . . . What You Choose to Eat Is Killing Our Planet*

Timothy Pachirat, *Every Twelve Seconds: Industrialized Slaughter and the Politics of Sight*

Steven Pinker, *The Better Angels of Our Nature: Why Violence Has Declined*

Steven Pinker, *Enlightenment Now: The Case for Reason, Science, Humanism, and Progress*

Jennifer Skiff, *Rescuing Ladybugs: Inspirational Encounters with Animals That Changed the World*

Rebecca Solnit, *Hope in the Dark: Untold Histories, Wild Possibilities*

Colin Spencer, *The Heretic's Feast: A History of Vegetarianism*

Tristram Stuart, *The Bloodless Revolution: A Cultural History of Vegetarianism from 1600 to Modern Times*

Will Tuttle, *The World Peace Diet: Eating for Spiritual Health and Social Harmony*

Frans de Waal, *Are We Smart Enough to Know How Smart Animals Are?*

# ENDNOTES

## Introduction

1. Mary Lou Randour, "Including Animal Cruelty as a Factor in Assessing Risk and Designing Interventions." Conference Proceedings, Persistently Safe Schools, The National Conference of the Hamilton Fish Institute on School and Community Violence, Washington, DC, 2004.

## SECTION ONE

### Chapter One: "Don't Tell Me. I Don't Want to Know": Blissful Ignorance and Willful Blindness

1. Margaret Heffernan, *Willful Blindness: Why We Ignore the Obvious at Our Peril* (New York: Bloomsbury USA, 2012), 3.
2. Melanie Joy, "Speaking Truth to Power: Understanding the Dominant, Animal-Eating Narrative for Vegan Empowerment and Social Transformation." One Green Planet, 2013, https://www.onegreenplanet.org/animalsandnature/speaking-truth-to-power-understanding-the-dominant-animal-eating-narrative-for-vegan-empowerment-and-social-transformation/.
3. Leon Festinger, *A Theory of Cognitive Dissonance* (Stanford: Stanford University Press, 1957).
4. "Per Capita Consumption of Poultry and Livestock, 1965 to Estimated 2018, in Pounds," National Chicken Council, last updated March 21, 2019, https://www.nationalchickencouncil.org/about-the-industry/statistics/per-capita-consumption-of-poultry-and-livestock-1965-to-estimated-2012-in-pounds/.

5. A. W. Speedy, "Global Production and Consumption of Animal Source Foods," *Journal of Nutrition* 133, no. 11S2 (November 2003): 4048–53, https://doi.org/10.1093/jn/133.11.4048S.

6. "Pet Industry Market Size and Ownership Statistics," American Pet Products Association, accessed May 9, 2019, http://www.americanpetproducts.org/press_industrytrends.asp.

7. "Results from a Recent Survey of American Consumers," American Society for the Prevention of Cruelty to Animals and Lake Research Partners, June 29, 2016, https://www.aspca.org/sites/default/files/publicmemo_aspca_labeling_fi_rev1_0629716.pdf.

8. Nico Pitney, "Revolution on the Animal Farm," *HuffPost,* updated September 23, 2016, http://www.huffingtonpost.com/entry/farm-animal-rights-revolution_us_577304f6e4b0352fed3e5b16.

9. Steve Loughnan, Brock Bastian, and Nick Haslam, "The Psychology of Eating Animals," *Current Directions in Psychological Science* 23, no. 2 (April 2014): 104, https://doi.org/10.1177/0963721414525781.

10. Loughnan, Bastian, and Haslam, "The Psychology of Eating Animals," 105.

11. Boyka Bratanova, Steve Loughnan, and Brock Bastian, "The Effect of Categorization as Food on the Perceived Moral Standing of Animals," *Appetite* 57, no. 1 (August 2011): 193–96, https://doi.org/10.1016/j.appet.2011.04.020.

12. Jeanette Settembre, "This Is the Insane Amount Millennials Are Spending on Fitness." *MarketWatch*, January 21, 2018, https://www.marketwatch.com/story/this-is-the-insane-amount-millennials-are-spending-on-fitness-2018-01-21.

13. The US Burden of Disease Collaborators, "The State of US Health, 1990–2016: Burden of Diseases, Injuries, and Risk Factors Among US States." *JAMA* 319, no. 14 (April 10, 2018): 1444–72, https://doi.org/10.1001/jama.2018.0158.

14. Sandra Galea, "America Spends the Most on Healthcare but Isn't the Healthiest Country." *Fortune*, May 24, 2017.

15. Stanley Cohen, *States of Denial: Knowing About Atrocities and Suffering.* (Cambridge, UK: Polity Press), 89–91.

16. Festinger, *A Theory of Cognitive Dissonance*, 30.

17. Heffernan, *Willful Blindness*, 54.

18. Heffernan, *Willful Blindness,* 84.

19. "StarKist's Charlie the Tuna," *Suicide Blog*, January 17, 2007, http://suicidefood.blogspot.com/2007/01/starkists-charlie-tuna.html.

20. United Egg Producers, "Animal Husbandry Guidelines for U.S. Egg-Laying Flocks," 2017, https://uepcertified.com/wp-content/uploads/2017/11/2017 -UEP-Animal-Welfare-Complete-Guidelines-11.01.17-FINAL.pdf.

21. Larry Sadler, Anna K. Johnson, and Suzanne T. Millman, "Alternative Euthanasia Methods to Manually Applied Blunt Force Trauma for Piglets Weighing Up to 12 Pounds," *Pork Information Gateway,* November 14, 2014, http:// porkgateway.org/resource/alternative-euthanasia-methods-to-manually-applied -blunt-force-trauma-for-piglets-weighing-up-to-12-pounds.

22. Heffernan, *Willful Blindness*, 247.

## Chapter Two: The Awakening: The Epiphany That Changes Everything

1. Timothy Pachirat, *Every Twelve Seconds: Industrialized Slaughter and the Politics of Sight* (New Haven: Yale University Press, 2013), 160.

2. Timothy Pachirat, "Working Undercover in a Slaughterhouse," interview by Avi Solomon, *Boing Boing*, March 8, 2012, https://boingboing.net/2012/03/08 /working-undercover-in-a-slaugh.html.

3. "Animal Farmers Going Vegan: Moving Quotes from Former Animal Agriculture Workers." *Last Chance for Animals* (blog), February 13, 2018, https:// www.lcanimal.org/index.php/blog/entry/animal-farmers-going-vegan-moving -quotes-from-former-animal-agriculture-workers-1.

4. Ashley Capps, "Former Meat and Dairy Farmers Who Became Vegan Activists," Free from Harm, November 4, 2014, https://freefromharm.org/animal -products-and-ethics/former-meat-dairy-farmers-became-vegan-activists.

5. Howard Lyman, "Straight Talk from a Former Cattleman," interview by Catherine Clyne, *Satya*, September 2006, http://www.satyamag.com/sept06/lyman .html.

6. Susana Romatz, "My Journey from 'Humane' Dairy Farmer to Vegan Cheese Maker," Humane Facts, March 6, 2017, http://humanefacts.org/from-humane -dairy-farmer-to-vegan-cheese-maker.

7. Capps, "Former Meat and Dairy Farmers Who Became Vegan Activists."

8. Carmen Lichi, "Former Dairy Farmer Tells How the Job Turned Her Vegan," *Woman's Day*, August 16, 2017, https://www.nowtolove.co.nz/health/diet -nutrition/farming-made-me-a-vegan-33880.

# SECTION TWO

## Staying Vegan

1. Faunalytics, "A Summary of Faunalytics' Study of Current and Former Vegetarians and Vegans," Faunalytics, February 24, 2016, https://faunalytics.org/a-summary-of-faunalytics-study-of-current-and-former-vegetarians-and-vegans.

## Stage One: Bearing Witness: Compassion Fatigue, Self-Care, and the Voracious Consumption of Information

1. Che Green, "Animal Advocacy by Numbers," Faunalytics, July 15, 2016, https://faunalytics.org/animal-advocacy-by-numbers.

2. "Reducing Suffering in Fisheries," Fish Count UK, accessed May 10, 2019, http://fishcount.org.uk.

3. "By the Numbers: GHG Emissions by Livestock," Food and Agriculture Organization of the United Nations, September 26, 2013, http://www.fao.org/news/story/en/item/197623/icode.

4. "Meat Eater's Guide to Climate Change and Health," Environmental Working Group, 2011, https://www.ewg.org/meateatersguide/interactive-graphic/water/.

5. "The USDA's War on Wildlife," Predator Defense, accessed May 10, 2019, http://www.predatordefense.org/USDA.htm.

6. Natural Resources Conservation Service, "Animal Manure Management," United States Department of Agriculture, December 1995, https://www.nrcs.usda.gov/wps/portal/nrcs/detail/null/?cid=nrcs143_014211.

7. "Discards and Bycatch in Shrimp Trawl Fisheries," Food and Agriculture Organization of the United Nations, accessed May 10, 2019, http://www.fao.org/docrep/W6602E/w6602E09.htm.

8. Sergio Margulis, "Causes of Deforestation of the Brazilian Amazon," *World Bank Working Paper* (22), 2004, World Bank, Washington, DC, http://documents.worldbank.org/curated/en/758171468768828889/pdf/277150PAPER0wbwp0no1022.pdf.

9. Lydia Zuraw, "2015 in Review: Animal Antibiotics," *Food Safety News*, December 28, 2015, http://www.foodsafetynews.com/2015/12/2015-in-review-animal-antibiotics/#.Ww7quFMvygB.

10. Michael Klaper, "Diet, Arthritis and Autoimmune Diseases," *Michael Klaper, M.D.* (blog), April 19, 2018, https://www.doctorklaper.com/diet-arthritis-autoimmune.

11. Jay Gordon, "Milk: Does It Really Do a Body Good?" *Jay Gordon, M.D.* (blog), February 23, 2010, http://drjaygordon.com/health-concerns/dairy-2.html.

12. Physicians Committee for Responsible Medicine, "Processed Meat: There Is No Safe Amount of Processed Meat," accessed May 10, 2019, http://www.pcrm.org /health/cancer-resources/diet-cancer/facts/meat-consumption-and-cancer-risk.

13. Joel Fuhrman, "Animal Products, the Microbiome, and Heart Disease," *Dr. Fuhrman* (blog), June 1, 2017, https://www.drfuhrman.com/library/eat -to-live-blog/143/animal-products-the-microbiome-and-heart-disease.

14. Compassion Fatigue Awareness Project, 2017, http://www.compassionfatigue .org.

15. Olga M. Klimecki, Susanne Leiberg, Claus Lamm, and Tania Singer. "Functional Neural Plasticity and Associated Changes in Positive Affect After Compassion Training," *Cerebral Cortex* 23, no. 7 (July 2013): 1552–61, https://doi .org/10.1093/cercor/bhs142.

16. Adam Hoffman, "When Empathy Hurts, Compassion Can Heal," *Greater Good*, August 22, 2013, https://greatergood.berkeley.edu/article/item/when _empathy_hurts_compassion_can_heal.

17. Sarah R. Hoffman, Sarah F. Stallings, Raymond C. Bessinger, and Gary T. Brooks. "Differences Between Health and Ethical Vegetarians: Strength of Conviction, Nutrition Knowledge, Dietary Restriction, and Duration of Adherence." *Appetite* 65 (June 1, 2013): 139–44. https://doi.org/10.1016/j.appet .2013.02.009.

18. Christine Carter, "Meditating with Kids," *Greater Good*, April 8, 2013, https:// greatergood.berkeley.edu/article/item/meditating_with_kids.

## Stage Two: Guilt, Regret, and Remorse: Finding Peace and Choosing Self-Forgiveness

1. "regret, n." OED Online, Oxford University Press, accessed December 6, 2018, http://www.oed.com/view/Entry/161391?isAdvanced=false&result=1&rskey =R4peZZ&.

2. "remorse, n." OED Online, Oxford University Press, accessed December 6, 2018, http://www.oed.com/view/Entry/162286?result=1&rskey=1zzRfZ&.

3. "forgive, v." OED Online, Oxford University Press, accessed November 30, 2018, http://www.oed.com/view/Entry/73337?result=1&rskey=moX8iy&.

## Stage Three: Coming Out Vegan: Explaining the V-Word to Family, Friends, and Yourself

1. Erving Goffman, *Stigma: Notes on the Management of Spoiled Identity* (New York: Simon & Schuster, 2009).

2. James O. Prochaska and Wayne F. Velicer, "The Transtheoretical Model of Health Behavior Change," *American Journal of Health Promotion* 12, no. 1 (May 5, 1997): 38–48, https://pdfs.semanticscholar.org/d8d1/915aa556ec4ff962 efe2a99295dd2e8bda89.pdf.

## Stage Four: Evangelism and Fundamentalism: Knowing the Difference Between Enthusiasm and Zealotry

1. Nathaniel M. Lambert, A. Marlea Gwinn, Roy F. Baumeister, et. al. "A Boost of Positive Affect: The Perks of Sharing Positive Experiences," *Journal of Social and Personal Relationships* 30, no. 1 (August 9, 2012): 24–43, https://doi .org/10.1177/0265407512449400.

2. Shahram Heshmat, "Why Do We Remember Certain Things, But Forget Others?," *Psychology Today,* October 8, 2015, https://www.psychologytoday.com/us /blog/science-choice/201510/why-do-we-remember-certain-things-forget-others.

3. Julia A. Minson and Benoît Monin, "Do-Gooder Derogation: Disparaging Morally Motivated Minorities to Defuse Anticipated Reproach," *Social Psychology and Personality Science* 3, no. 2 (July 18, 2011): 200–207, https://doi .org/10.1177/1948550611415695.

4. "fundamentalist, n. and adj."OED Online Oxford University Press, accessed November 6, 2018, http://www.oed.com/view/Entry/56739998?redirected From=fundamentalist.

5. Robert A. Denemark, "Fundamentalism and Globalization, *Oxford Research Encyclopedia of International Studies,* March 2010, https://dx.doi.org/10.1093 /acrefore/9780190846626.013.400.

6. Tobias Leenaert, *The Vegan Strategist* (blog), http://veganstrategist.org/.

## Stage Five: The Angry Vegan: Dispelling the Stereotype and Understanding Its Roots

1. "How Anger Affects the Brain and Body," National Institute for the Clinical Application of Behavioral Medicine, accessed May 10, 2019, https://www .nicabm.com/how-anger-affects-the-brain-and-body-infographic.

2. Glen Rein, Mike Atkinson, and Rollin McCraty, "The Physiological and Psychological Effects of Compassion and Anger, *Journal of Advancement in Medicine* 8, no. 2 (Summer 1995): 87–105, https://www.heartmath.org/research/research-library/basic/physiological-and-psychological-effects-of-compassion-and-anger/.

3. "Psychological Stress and Cancer," National Cancer Institute, reviewed December 10, 2012, https://www.cancer.gov/about-cancer/coping/feelings/stress-fact-sheet.

4. Michael O. Schroeder, "The Physical and Mental Toll of Being Angry All the Time," *U.S. News & World Report,* October 26, 2017, https://health.usnews.com/wellness/mind/articles/2017-10-26/the-physical-and-mental-toll-of-being-angry-all-the-time.

5. Tel Aviv University, "Why Cry? Evolutionary Biologists Show Crying Can Strengthen Relationships," *Science Daily,* September 7, 2009, https://www.sciencedaily.com/releases/2009/08/090824141045.htm.

6. Joan Halifax. "Quote of the Week: Roshi Joan Halifax." *The Jizo Chronicles* (blog), August 30, 2010. https://jizochronicles.com/2010/08/30/quote-of-the-week-roshi-joan-halifax-2/.

## Stage Six: Finding Your Tribe: Embracing Your Identity, Building Community, and Feeling a Sense of Belonging

1. R. F. Baumeister and M. R. Leary, "The Need to Belong: Desire for Interpersonal Attachments as a Fundamental Human Motivation," *Psychological Bulletin* 117, no. 3 (May 1995): 497–529, https://doi.org/10.1037/0033-2909.117.3.497.

2. Naomi I. Eisenberger, "The Neural Bases of Social Pain: Evidence for Shared Representations with Physical Pain." *Psychosomatic Medicine* 74, no. 2 (February 2012): 126–35, https://doi.org/10.1097/PSY.0b013e3182464dd1.

3. Faunalytics, "A Summary of Faunalytics' Study of Current and Former Vegetarians and Vegans," Faunalytics, February 24, 2016, https://faunalytics.org/a-summary-of-faunalytics-study-of-current-and-former-vegetarians-and-vegans.

4. Elise Amel, Christie Manning, Britain Scott, and Susan Koger. "Beyond the Roots of Human Inaction: Fostering Collective Effort Toward Ecosystem Conservation." *Science* 356, no. 6335 (April 21, 2017): 275–79, https://doi.org/10.1126/science.aal1931.

5. Tobias Leenaert, "Why Most People Eat Meat," *The Vegan Strategist* (blog), July 25, 2016, http://veganstrategist.org/2016/07/25/why-most-people-eat-meat.

6. Amel, Manning, Scott, and Kroger, "Beyond the Roots of Human Inaction."

7. Faunalytics, "A Summary of Faunalytics' Study of Current and Former Vegetarians and Vegans."

8. "Find Out How Many Vegans There Are in Great Britain," *The Vegan Society* (blog), Tuesday, May 17, 2016, https://www.vegansociety.com/whats-new/news/find-out-how-many-vegans-are-great-britain.

9. Joanna Young, Kip Johnson, and Jamie McCarthy, "And All the Men We Saw Today," University of Southampton, *Man Food*, accessed May 10, 2019, http://generic.wordpress.soton.ac.uk/man-food/wp-content/uploads/sites/298/2017/10/and-all-the-men-programme-notes.pdf.

10. Paul Rozin, Julia M. Hormes, Myles S. Faith, and Brian Wansink. "Is Meat Male? A Quantitative Multi-Method Framework to Establish Metaphoric Relationships." *Journal of Consumer Research* 39, no. 3 (October 2012): 629–43. https://papers.ssrn.com/sol3/papers.cfm?abstract_id=2473793.

11. Baumeister and Leary, "The Need to Belong."

12. Faunalytics, "A Summary of Faunalytics' Study of Current and Former Vegetarians and Vegans."

## Stage Seven: Finding Your Voice: How to Talk to a Hunter (Or Anyone Else with Whom You Disagree)

1. Stephen Mitchell, *Tao Te Ching: A New English Version* (New York: Harper Collins, 1991).

2. Jonathan Wise and Daniel Vennard, "It's All in a Name: How to Boost the Sales of Plant-Based Menu Items," World Resources Institute's Better Buying Lab, https://www.wri.org/news/its-all-name-how-boost-sales-plant-based-menu-items.

3. Candice Choi, "'Plant-Based' Replaces 'V-Words' to Appeal to Carnivores," *Christian Science Monitor,* August 2018, https://www.csmonitor.com/The-Culture/Food/2018/0824/Plant-based-replaces-v-words-to-appeal-to-carnivores.

4. "Consumer Trends in the Food and Beverage Industry," Morning Consult, accessed May 10, 2019, https://morningconsult.com/wp-content/uploads/2018/05/Morning-Consult-Consumer-Trends-In-The-Food-and-Beverage-Industry.pdf; James Tennent, "Nothing Is Less Appealing Than Vegan Food, Survey Finds," May 24, 2018, https://www.newsweek.com/nothing-less-appealings-vegan-food-survey-finds-942907.

5. Elaine Watson, "'Plant-Based' Plays Way Better than 'Vegan' with Most Consumers," *Food Navigator,* April 19, 2018, https://www.foodnavigator-us.com/Article/2018/04/19/Plant-based-plays-way-better-than-vegan-with-most-consumers-says-Mattson.

## Stage Eight: Stretching Your Comfort Zones: Expansion of Awareness and Skills

1. Margaret Heffernan, *Willful Blindness: Why We Ignore the Obvious at Our Peril* (New York: Bloomsbury USA, 2012).
2. Faunalytics, "A Summary of Faunalytics' Study of Current and Former Vegetarians and Vegans," Faunalytics, February 24, 2016, https://faunalytics.org/a-summary-of-faunalytics-study-of-current-and-former-vegetarians-and-vegans.
3. Cynthia Radnitza, Bonnie Beezholdb, and Julie DiMatteoa, "Investigation of Lifestyle Choices of Individuals Following a Vegan Diet for Health and Ethical Reasons," *Appetite* 90 (July 2015) 31–36, https://doi.org/10.1016/j.appet.2015.02.026.

## Stage Nine: Finding Your Place: Advocacy and Activism

1. Linda Tyler, "Lentil Loaf? Yuck! Increasing the Appeal of Plant-Based Dishes," Faunalytics, September 19, 2018, https://faunalytics.org/lentil-loaf-yuck-increasing-the-appeal-of-plant-based-dishes.
2. Greg Walton, Neil Malhotra, and Thomas Robinson, "Menu Messaging to Reduce Meat Consumption," Stanford Woods Institute for the Environment (2017), https://woods.stanford.edu/research/funding-opportunities/environmental-venture-projects/menu-messaging-reduce-meat-consumption.
3. Rebecca Solnit, *Hope in the Dark: Untold Histories, Wild Possibilities* (Chicago: Haymarket Books, 2016)
4. Steven Pinker, "Wielding Data Against Doom and Gloom," interview by Colleen Walsh, *Harvard Gazette*, February 27, 2018, https://news.harvard.edu/gazette/story/2018/02/harvards-pinker-makes-case-for-human-progress-in-new-book/.
5. Solnit, *Hope in the Dark.*
6. "What Is Gratitude?" *Greater Good Magazine*, accessed May 10, 2019, https://greatergood.berkeley.edu/topic/gratitude/definition#why_practice.
7. George Lakoff, "In Politics, Progressives Need to Frame Their Values," interview by Mark Karlin, *Truthout*, November 29, 2014, https://georgelakoff.com/2014/11/29/george-lakoff-in-politics-progressives-need-to-frame-their-values/.
8. Drew Desilver, "Despite Concerns about Global Democracy, Nearly Six in Ten Countries Are Now Democratic," Pew Research Center, December 16, 2017, http://www.pewresearch.org/fact-tank/2017/12/06/despite-concerns-about-global-democracy-nearly-six-in-ten-countries-are-now-democratic/.
9. Solnit, *Hope in the Dark.*

# ABOUT THE AUTHOR

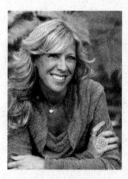

Colleen Patrick-Goudreau's compassionate living philosophy is propelling plant-based eating into the mainstream and forever changing how we regard animals.

A recognized expert and thought leader on the culinary, social, ethical, and practical aspects of living compassionately and healthfully, Colleen Patrick-Goudreau is a speaker, cultural commentator, podcaster, and award-winning author of seven books, including the bestselling *The Joy of Vegan Baking*, *The Vegan Table*, *Color Me Vegan*, *Vegan's Daily Companion*, *On Being Vegan*, and *The 30-Day Vegan Challenge*. She is an acclaimed speaker and beloved host of the inspiring podcast *Food for Thought*, which was voted Favorite Podcast by *VegNews* magazine readers several years in a row. She launched a spin-off podcast called *Animalogy* about the animal-related words and expressions we use every day and how they affect and reflect our treatment of animals. She is also the cofounder of East Bay Animal PAC, a political action committee that works with government officials on animal issues in the San Francisco Bay Area, and she volunteers as a "kitty cuddler" with Maine Coon Adoptions.

Colleen shares her message of compassion and wellness on national and regional TV and radio programs, including on "Good Day Sacramento" and as a monthly contributor on National Public Radio (KQED). She has appeared on the Food Network, CBS, PBS, and FOX; interviews with her have been featured on NPR, *Huffington Post,* and *U.S. News & World Report;* and her recipes have been featured on Epicurious.com and Oprah.com. Colleen lives in Oakland, California, with her husband, David, and two cats, Charlie and Michiko.